LIVINGSTON IMMUNOTHERAPY

THE TREATMENT OF CHRONIC, IMMUNE-DEFICIENT & AUTOIMMUNE DISEASES

Arthritis
Cancer
Chronic Fatigue Syndrome
Lupus
Scleroderma

By

ARTHUR DOUGLASS ALEXANDER III

© 2002, 2003 by Arthur Douglass Alexander III.
All rights reserved.

No part of this book may be reproduced, stored in a retrieval system, or transmitted by any means, electronic, mechanical, photocopying, recording, or otherwise, without written permission from the author.

ISBN: 1-4107-4013-7 (e-book)
ISBN: 1-4107-4012-9 (Paperback)

This book is printed on acid free paper.

1stBooks - rev. 04/23/03

CONTENTS

Dedication vii

Acknowledgements ix

Introduction xiii

1. The Life and Works of Dr. Virginia Wuerthele-Caspe Livingston, M.D. 1

2. The Microbiology and Immunology of Cancer - The Role of Mycobacteria 9

3. Mycobacteria in Cardiovascular Disease 24

4. The Livingston Foundation Medical Center Clinical Program 31

5. Clinical Treatment Program 37

6. The Nutritional Program 41

7. The Psychological Support Program 47

Summary 58

Appendix the Cookbook 61

Bibliography 156

Suggested Readings 164

About the Author 165

"All reproductive life, whether of the fetus in utero or of the cancer cell, is controlled by Chorionic Gonadotropin (CG). It is the hormone of life, and the hormone of death."

-Dr. Virginia Livingston, M.D. (1906-1990)

DEDICATION

Dedicated to Julie Anne Wagner, only daughter of Dr. Virginia Livingston, whose faith, courage and dedication have enabled her to sustain her mother's legacy of innovative, life-saving immunotherapies at the Livingston Foundation Medical Center.

ACKNOWLEDGEMENTS

Arthur Douglass Alexander gives special acknowledgement to the following friends and colleagues whose contributions have played such an important role in the creation of *"Livingston Immunotherapy"*:

Virginia Alexander, my devoted wife and helpmate who spent many hours researching the literature, making editorial suggestions and tirelessly proofing the manuscript,

Robert F. Barrett, Ph.D., former Executive Director and Staff Psychologist of the Livingston Foundation Medical Center,

Ana Maria Canales, author of *"The Cookbook"* for the Livingston Foundation who helped the author coordinate his work with both the Livingston Foundation and the Medical Center, and whose abridged work appears as an appendix,

Special Thanks: Anne Carr, for her invaluable editing assistance in the development of the final copy.

Chris Christenson, Ph.D., R.N., Staff Psychologist, Group Facilitator and Nursing Supervisor,

The late Kenneth C. Forror, M.D., former Medical Director, Livingston Foundation Medical Center,

Patricia M. Huntley, former longtime assistant to Dr. Virginia Livingston,

Mark Henri LaBeau, D.O., Staff Physician of Livingston Foundation Medical Center,

Dan I. Magtire, M.D., Retired, former Staff Physician, Livingston Foundation Medical Center,

John J. Majnarich, Ph.D., President and Scientific Director of BioResearch Laboratories in Redmond, Washington, Director of Livingston Foundation and Scientific Consultant to Livingston Foundation Medical Center, close friend and colleague of the late Dr. Virginia Livingston, M.D., and co-holder with Dr. Livingston of several key patents in the field of cancer microbiology and immunotherapy,

Linda Parker, Administrator of Livingston Foundation Medical Center,

Thelma Sterling, Livingston Foundation Medical Center Laboratory Supervisor,

Julie Anne Wagner, President of the Livingston Foundation and Livingston Foundation Medical Center, whose unwavering friendship, dedication and generous support have given "Livingston Immunology" life and meaning,

Gary R. Wagner, Secretary of the Livingston Foundation, whose enthusiastic support, steady hand, wise counsel and insight in the management, direction and clinical research of the Medical Center have proven invaluable to the author in preparing this manuscript,

Janet L. Zuckerman, Staff Nutritionist of Livingston Foundation Medical Center, and

Lucy Ritter, LVN, Ruth Bever and Lois Hazelhurst, all long time employees who worked closely with Dr. Livingston, helped everyone transition after her death to continue and further the work of the Medical Center. Their ongoing dedication maintains our high standards of excellence.

INTRODUCTION

Cancer reaches into every family around the world; it spares no one. One person in the United States dies of this dreaded disease every minute, over 1,400 a day, and 550,000 a year. The conventional treatments - surgery, radiation and chemotherapy - offer no real assurance of cure, and the financial burden these place on the patients and their families is often devastating.

It is human nature for the cancer patient to believe and trust in his physician and in the accepted, approved practices of our medical institutions. However, with the advent and growing awareness of alternative and complementary medicine in recent years a growing number of cancer patients are seeking options favoring less traumatic, non-toxic, immune enhancing therapies.

Billions of dollars are spent each year researching new therapies for the prevention, treatment and cure of cancer. Thousands of dedicated researchers and clinicians are devoting their lives to the conquest of the disease. Some are working in well-funded, well-equipped laboratories. Others, equally qualified, are working with little money and poor equipment. There are pioneers who persist in the face of discouragement from the medical establishment, finding ways to use the natural disease-fighting mechanisms with which we have been blessed as the main line of defense against cancer.

The late Dr. Virginia Livingston, M.D. was one of the first and remains one of the most important of these pioneers. Dr. Livingston discovered that a microbial agent, a mycobacterium which she called Progenitor cryptocides, was the fundamental causative agent of all human and animal cancers. Based upon her brilliant research findings and clinical therapies, this book reveals how the PC microbe produces many different forms of cancer and how it shields and protects itself from recognition and destruction by our natural immune systems. It also offers the reader hope for protection against the onset of the disease and control of cancer and other chronic diseases using the non-toxic, immunological therapies available at the Livingston Foundation Medical Center in San Diego, California.

THE LIFE AND WORKS OF DR. VIRGINIA WUERTHELE-CASPE LIVINGSTON, M.D.

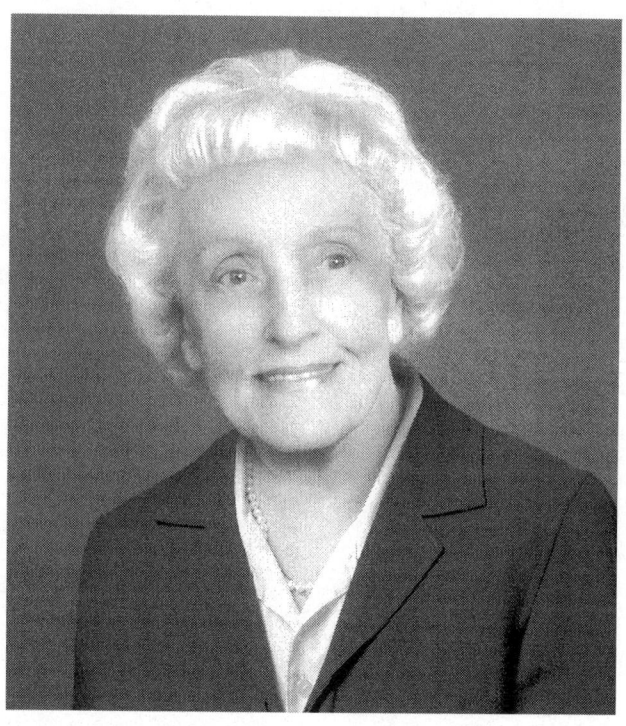

No description of the Livingston Foundation Medical Center and its outstanding immunotherapies for chronic diseases would be complete without citing the fascinating life and brilliant medical research of its founder, the late Virginia Livingston, M.D.

Dr. Virginia, as she liked to be called, was herself the daughter of a physician. She attended Vassar College and went on to graduate from Bellevue Medical College of New York University in 1936. Her residency was served in the infectious disease section of a New York prison hospital, where she worked with prostitutes infected with venereal diseases. Virginia later stated, "My preconceived notions of the prostitute underwent rapid reevaluation, and I developed great compassion for these women, often diseased and discarded by society." For the first time she used an instrument which would later play an important role in her cancer research studies—the darkfield microscope.

During the Second World War, Dr. Virginia worked as an industrial physician, screening job applicants at Western Electric. When she and her late husband, Dr. Joseph Caspe, a noted biochemist, adopted a baby, she took a part-time job as a school doctor in Newark, New Jersey.

One day a school nurse asked her to examine a skin disease with which she had become infected. Dr. Virginia took skin scrapings, and because she had seen many cases of tuberculosis and leprosy at the hospital prison, she stained these samples with the same Ziehl-Neelsen stain used to identify the leprosy and tuberculosis mycobacteria. She found "an acid-fast microorganism that was neither the lepra nor the tubercle bacillus." She reasoned it was a new "sclerobacillus", the cause of scleroderma, a progressive hardening of the skin that involves body organs and can be fatal. She was able to treat the nurse with appropriate medications, and she went on to publish her findings on scleroderma. Her work was confirmed at the Brussels Pasteur Institute and in other research in the United States.

Dr. Virginia next began gathering tumor samples and found the same microbes in her samples that she had taken from the nurse's skin scrapings. When these microbes were cultured and injected into mice, many developed cancer or collagen disease such as scleroderma or lupus erythematosis. Again she published these findings[1] and through her work began a longstanding clinical research partnership with Eleanor Alexander-Jackson, PhD, a microbiologist at Cornell Medical College and Irene Diller, M.D., of the Institute for Cancer

---

[1] V.W.Caspe, M.D., E.Alexander-Jackson, Ph.D., J.A. Anderson, Ph.D., J. Hillier, Ph.D., R.M.Allen, D.Sc. and L.W. Smith, M.D., "Cultural Properties and Pathogenicity of Certain Microorganisms Obtained from Various Proliferative and Neoplastic Diseases", American Journal of Medical Sciences, Vol 220 (1950) 42-52.

Research in Philadelphia. Dr. Virginia was also able to culture the Rous chicken "virus" in the laboratory a fact which indicated it was not a true virus as viruses cannot be grown outside the living host. She came to believe that the Rous chicken "virus" and perhaps other cancer "viruses" were related to the same mycobacterium she had isolated and identified earlier. Further, she showed that the cultured Rous chicken "virus" could be transmitted to other avian species—the first indication that some of the known cancer "viruses" were merely filterable phases of a pleomorphic bacteria. She subsequently classified this pleomorphic (having many forms) cancer-causing mycobacterium as a member of the Actinomycetales order of microorganisms that includes leprosy and tuberculosis. She named it Progenitor cryptocides."[2] The name "Progenitor" reflected her belief that the organism was primordial, and the term "cryptocides" indicates it to be a "hidden killer." Dr. Virginia met with Dr. Peyton Rous to discuss her findings with which Rous concurred. He subsequently postulated that possibly 95% of the chickens in New

---

[2] V.W.-C. Livingston, M.D. and A.M. Livingston, M.D., "Demonstration of Progenitor Cryptocides in the blood of Patients with Collagen and Neoplastic Diseases" from Transactions of the New York Academy of Sciences, Series II, Vol. 34, No. 5 (1972) 433-453.

York were infected with this "virus" and made the transmissibility of chicken cancer the subject of his Nobel Prize lecture in 1966. Based on her discovery that the chicken cancer mycobacterium is not destroyed by cooking, thereafter Dr. Virginia cautioned her patients about the very real danger of contracting cancer from eating even well-cooked chicken and eggs.

In 1965, Drs. Virginia Livingston and Eleanor Alexander-Jackson published a paper[3] on their identification of myocardial vascular disease brought about by the Progenitor cryptocides mycobacterium. Their hope was to focus attention on the possible underlying involvement of the pleomorphic mycobacterial pathogens in cardiovascular disease as well as the cardiovascular implications of mycobacterial-caused diseases.

In 1972, following extensive studies of fresh blood from cancer and non-cancer patients by darkfield microscopy, Dr. Virginia developed a modern nomenclature for the pleomorphic nature of the Progenitor cryptocides (PC) mycobacteria commonly seen in blood.

---

[3] V.W.-C. Livingston, M.D. and E. Alexander-Jackson, Ph.D., "Mycobacterial Forms in Myocardial Vasular Disease." Journal of the American Women's Association, Vol. 20, No. 5 (1965) 449-452.

These "forms" had previously been observed but not described or had been passed off as meaningless bacterial contaminants.

These studies were important in two ways: first, they revealed that a single mycobacteria could change its shape and form, thereby disguising itself as any one of a number of microbes, and second, that it was possible to arrest the growth of this bacteria. In 1974, Dr. Virginia published a landmark paper[4] reporting her findings that the PC mycobacteria produced a growth hormone immunologically and chemically similar to the human hormone, chorionic gonadotropin (HCG). This hormone is produced during pregnancy by the fetus to protect against attack by the mother's immune system. In the same manner, the HCG produced by the Progenitor cryptocides mycobacteria shields it from recognition by the patient's immune system, allowing it to grow out of control. It was subsequently found that abscisic acid actually blocks HCG produced by the PC mycobacteria, thus inhibiting the PC growth cycle. This suggested to

---

[4] V.W.-C. Livingston, M.D. and A.M. Livingston, M.D., "Some Cultural, Immunological and Biochemical Properties of Progenitor Crytptocides'" Transactions of the New York Academy of Science, Series II, Vol. 36, No. 6 (1974) 569-582.

Dr. Virginia that there was an ultimate weapon in the fight against human cancer—an antigen that could block HCG production.

Based on Dr. Virginia's work, the Livingston Foundation Medical Center's treatment of the immune-deficient patient is based upon the premise that Progenitor cryptocides is the primary exciting agent in the cancer process, that this killer microbe is shielded from the human immune system by the growth hormone, HCG, and that antigens represent the most effective means for destroying bacterial diseases and cancer because they challenge and stimulate the body's natural immune system.

During the 1970's (based upon her earlier discovery that the PC microbe is closely related to the tuberculosis and leprosy mycobacterium) Dr. Virginia began using the anti-tubercular antigen, Bacillus Calmette-Guerin (BCG) as an effective vaccine for stimulating her patients' immune systems. She prepared a personal immune antigen for each patient. Along with a carefully designed nutritional program, a stress-reducing psychoneuroimmunology (mind-body) component and conventional medical modalities, these immune-stimulating antigens and adjuvants form the foundation of the Livingston immunological treatment program.

Virginia Livingston, M.D. died of a fatal heart attack in June, 1990, while vacationing in Europe with her daughter, Julie Anne Wagner. Julie and her husband, Gary, have maintained and are continuing Dr. Virginia's commitment to providing effective immunotherapies for the treatment of immune deficient diseases, including cancer, through the Livingston Foundation for Cancer Research and Related Diseases. The Foundation sponsors the Livingston Foundation Medical Center and its fine medical staff in San Diego, California.

THE MICROBIOLOGY AND IMMUNOLOGY OF CANCER - THE ROLE OF MYCOBACTERIA

Background

For most of the twentieth century, medical science has been unable to define the nature of cancer or determine how its malignant growth cycle is unleashed at the cellular level. Since cancer cells are actually normal cells in which the genetic DNA has been altered, the human immune system does not readily recognize these mutant cells which replicate out of control. Medical researchers have spent the last fifty years trying to understand the cause of this mutation and then to evaluate the effects of various therapies on diseased and normal cells. Orthodox medicine focuses on surgery, radiation and chemotherapy as the recommended therapies to be used in the treatment of cancer. These therapies, which are aimed at eradicating cancerous growths or cells, do not address the cause and, unfortunately, deplete, impair or destroy the body's natural disease-fighting immune system.

Consequently, the prognosis for such common cancers as those of the breast, prostate, lung and colon has not changed in the last two decades. However, the emerging concept of cancer treatment is to harness and strengthen the patient's own natural defense system, the immune system, to fight cancer from within.

The Immune System and Disease

The body's first and best line of defense against disease is its own immune system. Extremely complex in design and function, the body's immune system is one of the most profound miracles of life. The immune system protects the body from within against the by-products of its normal biochemical reactions and from without as its only defense against foreign substances and toxic agents, including bacteria, viruses and chemical toxins. It discriminates between what is part of the body and what is not, between friend and foe, between what can help you or harm you. A strong, well-operating immune system routinely destroys literally millions of disease-carrying organisms and harmful substances present at almost all times in our bodies. It also participates in the repair and healing process after an affliction has been eradicated. It is both guardian and physician for the natural miracle that is the human body. Without a strong immune system, our bodies could not withstand the hostile environment which surrounds us, and we would quickly perish in an onslaught of disease.

How The Immune System Functions

There are four important functional elements of this complex defense system: antibodies, granulocytes (or white cells), something called complement, and lymphocytes. Antibodies are protein substances in the blood, created by the body to attack and destroy foreign bodies called antigens. Antibody-antigen reactions are generally specific—an antigen (of a disease, bacteria, virus, or foreign substance) will initiate the production of an antibody which will only attack that specific antigen.

A newborn baby does not possess a mature immune system and therefore must rely on antibodies naturally provided by its mother to fight infections. As the baby matures, so does its immune system. When it is exposed to antigens such as scarlet fever or chicken pox, for example, the baby begins to create its own antibodies that attack and neutralize these invading organisms. This process is assisted by vaccinations. When the baby is vaccinated—immunized—against a specific disease, it is given an extremely small amount of the disease antigen, allowing the immune system to recognize the disease, form antibodies, and remain fortified against that specific disease antigen.

The second line of defense in the body's immune system is granulocytes, or granulated white cells. These cells are constantly on patrol, tirelessly searching the body for poisonous material that would harm it. When granulocytes identify an invader, they mobilize millions of immune cells that attack relentlessly until the invader has been destroyed. When the granulocytes are incapable of overcoming these invaders on their own, they call in powerful reinforcements called macrophages, which are larger, stronger white blood cells.

The third component of the body's immune system is called complement, a group of nine highly specialized proteins in our blood serum that are manufactured by the liver and called into action by the antibodies. Complement is extremely aggressive, and cannot differentiate between friend or foe, and will attack normal healthy cells as quickly as it will poisonous invaders. Complement therefore requires a guidance system which is provided by the antibodies. The antibodies attach a "marker" to each disease antigen thereby identifying it. Then they activate the nearest passing unit of complement. The first of the complement's nine proteins attaches to the marker on the antigen, signals the second unit of complement to attach to the cell wall of the agient. This process continues until the ninth unit of complement attaches to the antigen's cell wall, at which time, the invading cell is broken up and destroyed.

Lymphocytes are the fourth component of the immune system. They are the watchdogs of the system, constantly patrolling, searching for invaders and mobilizing the body's defenses. Lymphocytes are secreted by lymph nodes located throughout the body. They have no means of locomotion but are carried along in the blood stream through tissues and organs, muscles and skin. Eventually they will pass through a nearby lymph node and recycle through the body again and again. Unlike granulocytes, Lymphocytes continue to live for months and years, making their inspection patrols hundreds of times a day. The whole system is actually controlled by these lymphocytes.

When a bacterium enters the body, say through a cut on the finger or from stepping on a nail at the beach, the antibodies already existing in the immune system will attack it and prevent infection. If the infection has gained a foothold, the entire system will become mobilized to fight it. If a new invader appears, one that hasn't been in the body before, it will eventually encounter one of the circulating lymphocytes. The lymphocyte makes a print or copy of the invading antigen's marker and relays this information to the nearest lymph node. The lymph node, in turn, alerts the entire system, mobilizing antibodies to seek the new antigen's marker and destroy it.

Against especially tough invaders—viruses or parasites that may have strong protective shells around them (such as the cancer-causing Progenitor cryptocides mycobacterium microbe), we must assist the natural immune system to recognize these invaders by deshielding them with specially designed adjuvants so that the immune system's natural killer (NK) cells can recognize and destroy these microbes. This process is called "immunotherapy."

Immunotherapy and Bacterial Infection

Immunology is the science that deals with the phenomena and causes of immunity in the body, while "immunotherapy" encompasses the actual clinical treatment of disease by restoring and enhancing the body's natural defense mechanisms. Immunotherapy utilizes natural substances of biological origin, including natural nutritional supplements, and extracts or components of viruses and bacteria. These methods help the body to recognize its own mutant cancer cells, for example, and to produce specific antibodies which selectively attack, and genetically alter, or destroy the cancer cells.

Long advocated by the Livingston Foundation Medical Center and its founder, immunotherapy is finally gaining broad acceptance throughout the medical community as perhaps the most effective approach to the treatment of serious, chronic diseases. Perhaps we are all potential victims of cancer because we all have the cancer microbes in our bodies. Those of us with stronger immune systems keep the microbes in check. As the use of immunotherapy increases, so does the chance of overcoming debilitating or life-threatening afflictions such as cancer. In recognition of this potential, the National

Institutes of Health (NIH) have added an Office of Complementary and Integrative Medicine, and the National Cancer Institute (NCI) has stated that vaccines could prevent the initial development of cancer. Vaccines could also function therapeutically, says the Institute, to prevent the metastatic spread or recurrence of a tumor, thus playing a huge role in reducing the life-threatening potential of cancer.

In 1950, Dr. Virginia Livingston was successful in identifying and isolating a bacterial agent common to all forms of human and animal cancer—a mycobacterium closely related to that which causes tuberculosis and leprosy. She classified this cancer mycobacterium as a member of the Actinomycetales order of bacteria, calling it Progenitor cryptocides, or PC. Over the past fifty years since her discovery, prominent research has established links between certain bacterial and viral infections, inflammation and most cancers. Many investigators have reported the discovery of certain bacterial isolates from human and animal cancer tissue, as well as from the blood and urine of cancer hosts. Extensive evidence clearly linking the PC mycobacteria to cancer, carefully documented by Drs. Wuerthele-Caspe (Livingston), Jackson, et.al., was published in the prestigious

American Journal of Medicine Sciences in December of 1950. Later confirmatory studies were published in the annals and transactions of the New York Academy of Sciences in 1970 and 1972. Dr. Irene Diller of the Cancer Research Institute of Philadelphia reported that specific bacterial isolates injected into mice produced cancerous tumors.

Despite this convincing research, bacterial organisms have been generally ignored as a potential cause of cancer. The reason may lie in the evasive nature of organisms such as Progenitor cryptocides. They are masters of disguise. They take many different forms in the course of their growth and replication cycle (they are pleomorphic see figure 1), and these different forms mimic those of other, non-cancer causing strains of bacteria. They have been variously described as round, coccal forms, spores, spore sacs, straight and curved rods, and sometimes a fungi. Some investigators even claimed they, like viruses, would pass through fine microbiological filters. Frequently, these organisms were identified as Staphylococcus bacteria. However, careful study shows them to be cell wall deficient, which Staphylococcus bacteria are not. Neverthless, in spite of attempts to invalidate the findings of Dr. Livingston and others, extensive evidence remains linking these bacteria to cancerous human and animal tumors.

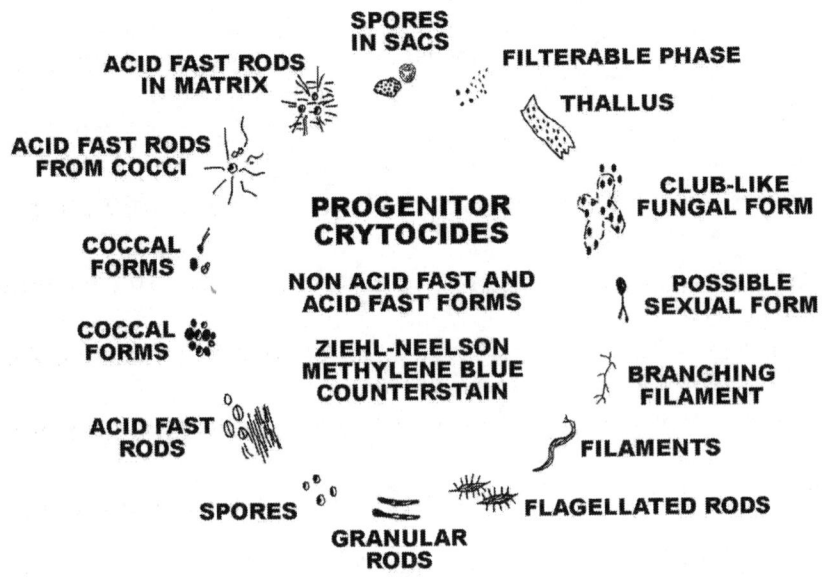

Figure 1: The Pleomorphic Forms of Progenitor Cryptocides Mycobacteria

The Universal Cancer Marker—HCG—The Reproductive Hormone

As stated earlier, cancer may be characterized as the uncontrolled, rapid growth of mutant cells which escape detection and destruction by the immune system and begin to invade healthy tissues. Many researchers now believe that cancer growth closely parallels fetal growth within the mother's womb. In addition to having the capacity for extremely rapid cell divisions—common to both cancer and fetal development—cancer cells appear to share the same mechanism by which an embryo avoids attack by its mother's immune system.

Human chorionic gonadotropin (HCG), the first hormone produced by the fertilized ovum to signal pregnancy, possesses a number of functions vital to the establishment and maintenance of pregnancy, and is produced in large quantities by the developing fetus. Fetal embryonic cells constitute a threat to the mother's immune system, which, if left unchecked, would in turn destroy its own offspring. During pregnancy, HCG coats the surface of the fetal cells and shuts down any attack by the mother's immune system. The fetus and the mother thereby strike a necessary balance in which the fetus is allowed to grow, while the mother's immune system remains effective throughout the rest of her body. HCG is not normally produced or found in non-pregnant women unless they have cancer. Unless they have cancer, men normally only produce HCG on the surface of sperm cells or in the testes.

By demonstrating that all cancer cells possess PC mycobacteria and that these mycobacteria produce HCG, Dr. Livingston showed that the HCG growth hormone also shields and protects cancer cells from recognition and attack by the body's immune system. The fact that most normal cells do not produce HCG suggests that an anti-HCG immunotherapy may offer a very specific means of treating cancer. Using different strategies, the therapy would help the body's natural defenses to overcome the barricades shielding the cancer cell. A number of scientists have come to believe that HCG represents an important clue for successfully treating cancer.

Because the PC microbe, in one of its many forms, looks like a plant fungus, Dr. Virginia reasoned that a botanical substance might block its growth and replication. As a result, she discovered that abscisic acid (a plant hormone called dormin, a retinoid or Vitamin A analog that produces dormancy in seeds) plays a major regulatory role in the production of the HCG growth hormone by the PC microbe. In other words, abscisic acid neutralizes production by the tumor or PC microbe of HCG. This, in turn, prevents the cancer cells from camouflaging themselves with HCG and allows the immune system to find and destroy them. This may be the reason that foods rich in Vitamin A analogs, the retinoids and abscisins, which may be derived from fresh vegetables appear to have a beneficial action in preventing and controlling cancer. As a result Dr. Virginia introduced a form of abscicic acid (which she named Cis-14) into her patients' diets to naturally treat a vitamin deficiency, and to stimulate their immune systems to control the growth of the PC mycobacteria. (see Figure 2)

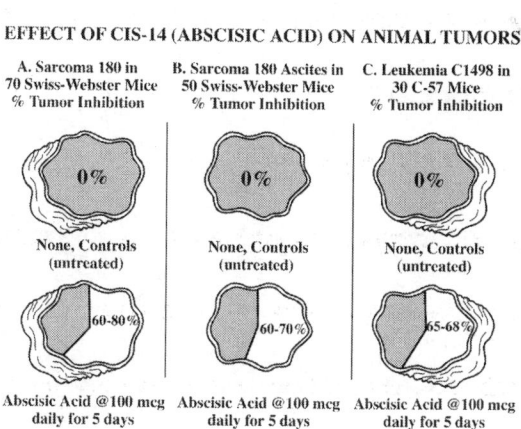

EFFECT OF CIS-14 (ABSCISIC ACID) ON ANIMAL TUMORS

A. Sarcoma 180 in 70 Swiss-Webster Mice % Tumor Inhibition — None, Controls (untreated) 0%; Abscisic Acid @ 100 mcg daily for 5 days 60-80%

B. Sarcoma 180 Ascites in 50 Swiss-Webster Mice % Tumor Inhibition — None, Controls (untreated) 0%; Abscisic Acid @ 100 mcg daily for 5 days 60-70%

C. Leukemia C1498 in 30 C-57 Mice % Tumor Inhibition — None, Controls (untreated) 0%; Abscisic Acid @ 100 mcg daily for 5 days 65-68%

Dr. Livingston's findings have been confirmed by numerous investigators in laboratories around the world, including Drs. Herman F. Acevedo and Malcolm Slifkin in 1976 at the Department of Laboratory Medicine of Allegheny General Hospital in Pittsburgh.[5] In 1992, Dr. Acevedo and his associates completed development of a new, more sensitive method for detecting cells that produce HCG. These findings were published in April 1992 in Cancer, the scientific journal of the American Cancer Society. Applying the new methodology to 74 different cancer cell lines, spanning fifteen different types of cancer, Acevedo and his team found all of them to be producing the HCG hormone. Dr. Acevedo's research confirmed the common link of HCG in cancer cell growth and the development of the human fetus. Currently Dr. Acevedo is continuing his work to determine the specific mechanisms which enable HCG to render a cell immunologically invisible.

As a result of the outstanding microbiological work by Drs. Livingston and Acevedo, a growing number of scientists and

---

[5] Acevedo, Hernan F., et al., "Human Chorionic Gonadotropin in Cancer Cell Systems," Press: Proc. Third International Symposium of the Detection and Prevention of Cancer, Ed. H.E. Nieburgs, Marcel Dekker, Inc., New York, NY, (1976).

clinicians have come to believe that HCG may be a prime target on cancer cells to which a variety of therapeutic agents and antigens should be directed. The editor of the American Cancer Society's journal, Cancer, asks, "Have we found the definitive cancer biomarker?" and concludes that the "beta" segment of HCG is "a key factor defining the metastatic phenotype (of cancer). Based on the work of Acevedo and his associates, we must continue to ask why reproduction and cancer are paradoxically inseparable."

Perhaps we can find the answer in Dr. Virginia Livingston's profound statement that: "All reproductive life, whether of the fetus or of the cancer cell, is controlled by Human Chorionic Gonadotropin (HCG). **It is the hormone of life, and the hormone of death.**

MYCOBACTERIA IN CARDIOVASCULAR DISEASE

In her book, <u>Cancer, A New Breakthrough</u>, Dr. Livingston wrote of her own life-threatening experience in 1962. "My heart appeared to stop…I had no pulse and became extremely weak…I told my husband I was having a serious heart attack, that I must leave my clinic and be taken to a nearby cardiologist in La Jolla."

Dr. Livingston barely survived that initial heart attack. After 10 days in the hospital, she was returned to her home, where, for the next two years, she required a full-time nurse-companion in attendance. As she slowly regained her strength, she began to explore her options for prevention of another attack. During this time she also reread many of her own scientific research papers on cancer and mycobacteria. She was struck by the fact that many of the research animals inoculated with the cancer causing mycobacterium, Progenitor cryptocides (PC), had also developed heart lesions. Baby mice born of infected mothers often died, and autopsies showed that their heart muscles had been destroyed by the same PC bacteria.

Dr. Livingston read reports by a number of clinical researchers in England who had found strange, microbial bodies in the hearts of patients who had died of coronary disease. Armed with this confirmation of her own observations, she turned to immunotherapy as the answer for her own recovery. She contacted her close friend and former colleague, Dr. Eleanor Alexander-Jackson, who offered to prepare a vaccine for Dr. Virginia according to the method developed in England. The vaccine was made by culturing dormant PC mycobacteria remaining in Dr. Virginia's system from a successfully treated cancer of the forehead. The vaccine effectively controlled the mycobacteria responsible for her heart attack and restored her heart muscle to health.

In 1965, Drs. Livingston and Alexander-Jackson wrote a paper[6] in which they proposed the theory that there are microbial bodies in the lesions of diseased hearts, and that these lesions are particularly numerous in the areas where blood vessels have ruptured. More recently, medical researchers are becoming aware that vessels in the heart rupture not because of cholesterol deposits on the inside, as was

---

[6] Virginia W.-C. Livingston, M.D. and Eleanor Alexander-Jackson, Ph.D., "Mycobacterial Forms in Myocardial Vascular Disease," Journal of the American Medical Women's Association, Vol. 20, No. 5, (May, 1965) 449-52.

previously thought, but because of disease of the tissues and muscles of the heart which support the vessels from the outside. This disease might be caused by microbial infection.

Drs. Livingston and Jackson were able to identify and demonstrate degenerative changes occurring in coronary heart disease in the presence of invasive mycobacterial parasites. Experimenting with animals, they found that lesions produced by these organisms affected not only the heart, but most of the other principal organs of the body. The two women then went on to study postmortem heart sections of six patients with coronary and aortic disease. Microscopic examination revealed:

1. Small, acid-fast bodies from these organisms in the loose, connective tissues around the small coronary vessels.
2. Cellular infiltration around the vessels and between the muscle fibers as well. These cells consisted predominantly of immune-system lymphocytes and mononuclear phagocytes laden in both the granular and coccobacillary forms of these organisms.

3   The presence of fibroblasts apparently stimulated by the presence of these organisms. In some areas, the normal muscle fibers or interstitial tissues appeared to be replaced by fibroblasts.

4   Numerous small, acid-fast cocci and coccobacilli where there had been an infarct (an obstruction in the coronary vessel caused by a thrombus or embolus).

5   Necrosis (localized death of tissue) of the blood vessels showing striking degeneration of the blood vessel walls and aorta with many changes brought about by hair-like filaments of the organisms.

6   Changes in the elastic layer of the aorta in which masses of these organisms proliferated together with polyhedral crystals resembling cholesterol.

7   Individual nuclei of the heart muscles that had been parisitized and replaced by small, acid-fast, bodies of the organism. The heart muscle fibers appeared to be in a state of gradual digestion and disintegration by both minute and larger acid-fast forms of the organisms.

This important work focused attention on the possible involvement of pleomorphic, mycobacterial pathogens, such as the Progenitor cryptocides cancer-causing mycobacterium in cardiovascular disease. In addition, leading clinical scientists have recently discovered that viruses, and particularly the Herpes family of viruses may be significantly involved in causing arterial disease and heart attacks. Dr. Joseph L. Melnick, a virologist at Baylor College of Medicine in Houston, suggested that the Herpes viruses may trigger coronary heart disease. He reasoned that many people are infected early in their lives with one or more the Herpes viruses which may remain dormant for years. Melnick found evidence that the cytomegalo virus (CMV), a member of the Herpes family, along with a fat-rich diet may initiate atherosclerosis by promoting plaque formation in the arterial walls.

In 1994, Drs. Stephen Epstein and Edith Speir of New York proposed a link between arterial disease and cancer—the p53, "anti-tumor" gene whose loss or inactivation may contribute to as many as 50% of all human cancers. In 1997 Dr. Epstein confirmed that in heart patients, the cytomegalo virus is responsible for blocking the action of this vital growth-limiting p53 protein which prevents excessive post-surgical tissue growth within arteries following angioplasty or coronary bypass surgery. When the cytomegalo virus combines with the p53 protein and blocks its normal function, the tissues at the surgical sites continue to grow. After eight to ten years the normal blood flow through these tissues is seriously constricted. In a similar fashion, the cytomegalo virus also inactivates p53 protein at tumor sites, allowing an unchecked growth of the cancerous tissue.

Once again, an important response to the invasion of cardiovascular tissue by mycobacteria and viruses may be immunotherapy. In the 1970's, Dr. Catherine Fabricant at Cornell College of Veterinary Medicine infected some chickens with an avian herpes virus. Though these test birds were fed a cholesterol-free diet, they developed a condition similar to human atherosclerosis. A second group of herpes-infected birds were fed a diet rich in cholesterol, which produced severe clogging of their arteries. A third group of test birds was vaccinated against the avian herpes virus, and subsequently fed a diet extremely rich in cholesterol. These birds were resistant to the development of fat-laden arteries. Through the immunization they had been protected from disease.

THE LIVINGSTON FOUNDATION MEDICAL CENTER CLINICAL PROGRAM

The success of the Livingston Foundation Medical Center in San Diego, California is based on a carefully researched and clinically proven therapeutic program. The program has been designed to restore and enhance the body's natural immune system and to empower the patient to fight effectively against the causes of serious, chronic and autoimmune diseases, including cancer. Since opening its doors in 1970, the Center has helped thousands of patients, many of whom have come to the Center in desperation, knowing their lives are threatened by a killer disease for which they have been told there is "no cure".

Most patients initially contact the Center by telephone or internet and receive an information packet about the Center's program. This packet includes a summary of the immunological protocols, a synopsis of the standard ten-day outpatient treatment program and a request for all medical information pertinent to the patient's current health status. If you enroll in the program as a patient, you will be encouraged to bring a companion. During the therapeutic program you and your companion will be instructed by the staff in the use and administration of medications and injections, the preparation of special foods essential to restoring and maintaining a healthy, immune-supportive nutritional program. You will also be taught the importance of psychological support and stress reduction techniques in your healing process.

The founder of the Center, Dr. Virginia Livingston, always received her patients with love, concern, medical expertise and reassurance. Today, the staff carries on her tradition. When you arrive at the center, you will know immediately that this is a place where everyone cares about your well-being and comfort.

After participating in an orientation with staff members, you will be asked to write out your medical history in as much detail as possible. You will be asked to supply the background of your family's medical history as well because diseases such as diabetes and cancer may have an hereditary component. You will then consult with a Center physician, who will share with you the total benefit of his knowledge and skill for the duration of your involvement with the

Center. Areas of non-medical concerns are also explored during this interview, for it is important to identify those stress factors and previously unsuccessful therapies which may have contributed to weakening your immune system.

After the interview, you will be given a thorough physical examination. Because they represent the accumulated knowledge of modern medicine, all conventional diagnostic techniques are employed. These include blood counts and chemistry, blood protein tests, urinalysis, determination of electrolyte balance, kinds, types and amounts of circulating antibodies, thyroid function, steroid levels, and radiological, diagnostic tests as indicated. If special procedures and tests are needed, you will be referred to one of the specialists in the San Diego area.

A clean-catch urine specimen will be obtained. It will be cultured for bacterial growth. The Progenitor cryptocides (PC) organisms will be identified, isolated and later used to prepare a Personal Immune Antigen (PIA). It is very important to determine the number and forms of these pleomorphic mycobactera and to follow their numbers after treatment. When necessary, microbial isolates are used to perform an antibiotic sensitivity test to determine whether antibiotics might be helpful to you.

The LFMC uses a very specialized tool, the darkfield microscope. While in this country, it has been used primarily as a research tool, in Europe it is a common instrument in the offices of many doctors who study and treat chronic diseases. With it your blood will be examined and the PC microbe may be seen circulating in your system. This provides a simple test for routinely monitoring the progress of the treatment.

In addition, you will be given a number of standard tests, including a host of tumor markers, which utilize specific proteins, to determine cancerous activity. Many clinical laboratories are now using tumor markers as key diagnostic tests for cancer. They provide non-invasive information about the amount of tumor present, and the degree of its advancement and activity.

The hope of the future may be in integrating immunotherapies with traditionally accepted methods of treatment. At LFMC, special attention is paid to evaluating the function of your immune system. Because of the size and complexity of the immune system, there is no perfect or comprehensive test to determine its health. Therefore, a series of tests is utilized, including darkfield microscopy, immune T-, B-, and NK cell studies. These analyze the body's populations of specialized types of lymphocytes, which are important in mounting an immune response to bacteria and disease. Tumor markers, proteins made by cancer cells, are measured to allow us to monitor the effectiveness of the immunotherapy.

The prevailing belief at LFMC is that cancer has a number of contributing causes including the Progenitor cryptocides mycobacterium, stress, environmental exposure to toxins and carcinogens, nutritional deficiencies and excesses, as well as genetic predisposition. Therefore, it makes good sense that the more comprehensive the approach to treatment, the better the outcome will be. LFMC's treatment programs are individualized for each patient to address as many factors as possible. Your program will be comprised of three major components. The first is the clinical treatment program emphasizing the use of antigens (vaccines) which enhance the ability of the depleted immune system to overcome disease. The second is the use of nutrition and nutrient supplements to further strengthen the natural immune system, and the third is psychological support and patient health counseling, which have evolved into the Center's psychoneuroimmunology (mind-body) component.

EFFECT OF e+ FACTOR ALONE & IMMUNE ANTIGEN VS. SARCOMA 180 IN 10 MICE

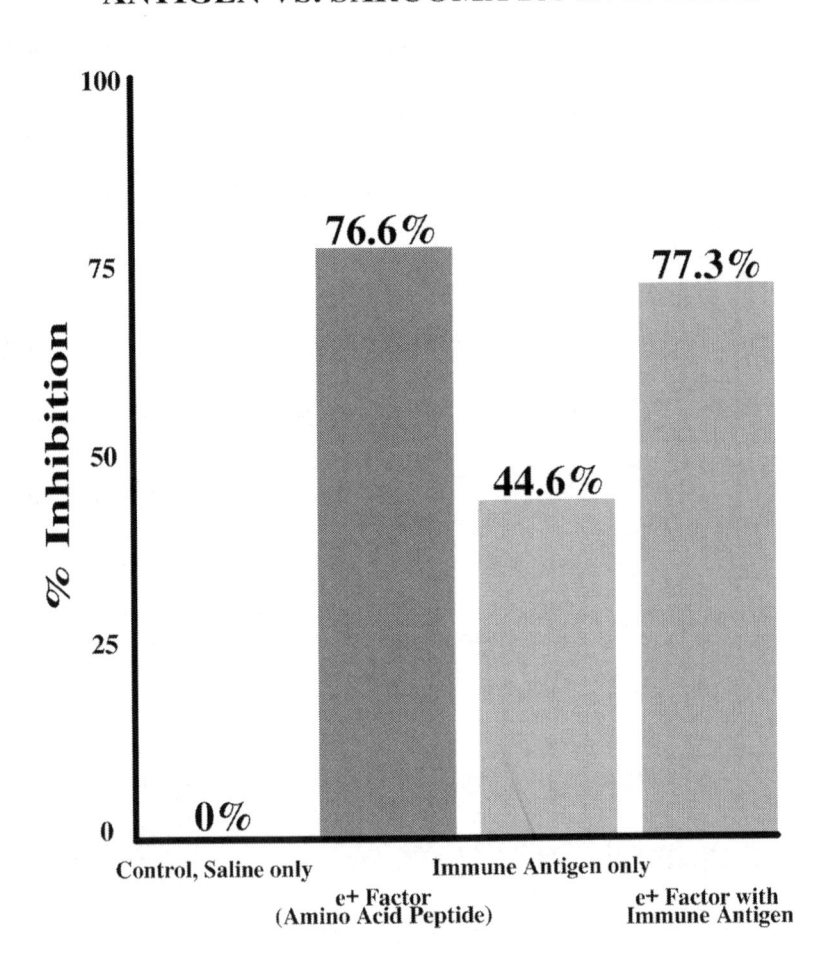

% Inhibition:
- Control, Saline only: 0%
- e+ Factor (Amino Acid Peptide): 76.6%
- Immune Antigen only: 44.6%
- e+ Factor with Immune Antigen: 77.3%

CLINICAL TREATMENT PROGRAM

Antigens and vaccines are the cornerstones of the Livingston clinical immunotherapy program, and are what makes it unique. A number of antigens are used to stimulate and enhance the patient's immune system including some cultured from the patient's own cells. Once scientists isolate and characterize an organism that causes a disease, they are often able to induce the immune system to produce specific antibodies that then attack the surface of the organism, either destroying it or rendering it incapable of reproducing. This is done by introducing a small amount of the actual organism or antigen into the patient's system. The immune system then mobilizes its forces to rid the body of the invading organism.

The primary induction and enhancement of the patient's immunity begins with the use of the Bacillus Calmette-Guerin (BCG) vaccine, while a personal immune antigen (PIA) is being prepared. BCG, a live tubercule bacillus and a close relative of Progenitor crytocides, has been found to be a powerful instrument with which to jump start the patient's natural immune system. The response usually starts within 24 hours. New patients may receive two to four BCG vaccinations during their initial two-week treatment. During this time a Personal Immune Antigen will be prepared to meet the specific needs of the patient. Because the PC organisms are excreted in the patient's urine, they can be cultured from a clean catch urine sample. They are then used to create the Personal Immune Antigen, which is again administered through the vaccination process.

Small, increasing doses of non-specific antigens including Gamma globulin may also be used. These adjuvants are useful in treating arthritis and controlling chronic recurrent infections such as colds, which lower the patient's resistance and tax the already weakened immune system. If a patient's white blood cell count is low, either because of chemotherapy or general wasting and malnutrition often associated with chronic disease, Custom Formula antigen will be used. It is a thymus-splenic-liver extract derived from disease-free sheep.

Should the darkfield microscope show an excess of bacterial forms in the patient's blood, antibiotics may become important. When the right antibiotic is selected and administered in standard doses, the tumors themselves also may diminish in size. Antibiotics, when appropriate, generally decrease the number of PC mycobacteria circulating in the blood. Frequently, ampicillin, septra, keflex, or cipro are used for varying periods of time; again depending on the darkfield microscopic blood analysis. Each case is carefully evaluated by blood examination and urine cultures, followed by frequent sensitivity tests to make certain a patient is not developing a resistance or an allergic reaction to the antibiotics.

Antioxidents, supplements and trace minerals may also be prescribed as indicated by the patient's extensive blood test panels. Many cancer patients are metabolizing intensely in their fight to rid their body of the disease, and many will become thyroid deficient in the process. Small doses of thyroid hormone may be needed to supplement the patient. Again, this regimen is determined by laboratory testing. Occasionally, suppressive hormones, such as tamoxifen, may be used for treating hormone-dependent tumors.

If you are a smoker, you will be required to stop when you enter treatment because tobacco is a proven carcinogen. Alcohol is also not allowed during your recovery process. The detoxification of alcohol puts a tremendous strain on the liver, which must be restored to peak performance in order to produce the enzymes necessary for the metabolism of Vitamin A and essential proteins—essential energy products. Upon leaving the Center you will be asked to avoid contact with all chemicals such as cleaning solutions, solvents, paint removers, insect sprays and other products which can seriously impair a weakened immune system.

THE NUTRITIONAL PROGRAM

Dr. Virginia Livingston wrote in 1984, "One of the most vital systems of the body that cannot be sustained by devitalized, dead food is the immune system." Today physicians and scientists around the world are realizing that the unwholesomeness and lack of nutritional value of our modern diets are responsible for the degeneration of our health. As a result of consuming imitation foods or "non-foods", we first undermine, then destroy, our resistance to disease. Poor nutrition sets the stage for serious chronic illness.

An enormous number of the foods we eat, including our meat and vegetables, have been frozen somewhere along the line—either in a refrigerated truck or railroad car, in the store, or in our own homes. Food can lose many of its natural nutrients in the freezing and defrosting process. Washing foods to remove surface contaminants and preservative chemicals unfortunately also removes many minerals and vitamins that are found in abundance on the skins and outer layers of fruits and vegetables. Consider further that insecticides on fruit, preservatives to keep bread fresh, additives to make tomatoes and beets redder, additives used in processing cheese, sweeteners in catsup and soft drinks, sugar in cereal and peanut butter (the list goes on and on) react with the remaining nutrients in our food to render the vitamins and minerals of little or no value.

Methods of cooking may also destroy the nutritional value of our food. Exposing food to hot grease, hot dry air, excessive heat or smoke—frying, broiling, charcoal broiling or oven roasting may not only destroy essential vitamins and minerals, but may also produce toxins that have been reported to be cancer-causing carcinogens.

Good nutrition is essential in maintaining and restoring a healthy, functional immune system. The majority of the cellular components that make up the immune system are comprised of proteins. We know the healthy immune system requires a steady intake of protein in order to manufacture its armies of specialized disease-fighting cells and antibodies. Proteins are made up of components called amino acids. There are 22 different amino acids which are arranged by the body in varying sequences to produce the required immune system proteins. Our bodies can normally synthesize many of these. However, there are eight amino acids, the essential amino acids, that cannot be synthesized and therefore must be derived from the food we eat. These are found scattered among certain plants and vegetables, or are derived in a more concentrated form from various animal sources.

Looking at animal sources first, we note a similarity between the ways that human biological systems and animal systems function. Animal protein is a rich, concentrated source of available components from which our bodies can readily draw and reestablish needed protein. However, animal protein may also contain toxins and other pollutants. It is a growth medium for microbes and bacteria, many of which are pathogenic and may include the Progenitor cryptocides mycobacterium. This raises a serious risk-benefit question. Is the benefit of having a rich source of animal protein available for the immune system worth the risk of burdening the body with toxins, pathogens and pollutants?

Animal protein is only as good as the health of the animal itself. The required government food inspection is inadequate since it is limited to gross inspection and does not involve microscopic examination of tissues except in rare cases. In the past it has been found that 25% of the cattle going to slaughter harbor a pathological infection by the PC mycobacterium. Chickens are a widely consumed source of protein, and their body temperature of 105 degrees eliminates many of the common pathogens such as staphylococcus. Unfortunately it also provides an ideal incubation environment for the PC mycobacteria. Since only about one in five million sheep have cancer, lamb, together with wild game and fresh fish from unpolluted waters provide excellent sources of protein for human consumption.

An alternative source of protein may be derived from plants, particularly from beans, whole grains, raw nuts, seeds and soy products as well as protein powders, many of which include concentrated greens. At first glance, the total protein count in plant sources may seem higher than in animals. However, in some plants the proportion of the essential amino acids may be more limited. Therefore, we must carefully select a variety of plant sources to provide the best bioavilability of protein for the human immune system, and particularly for one weakened by a debilitating chronic disease. Plants also provide a number of other nutrients, and, in their unrefined state, a generous amount of fiber. Fiber not only has an affinity for trapping toxins, pollutants, excess hormones and cholesterol, but also represents a food source for beneficial organisms that inhabit the body. The following are examples of topics that are discussed with our patients by our nutritional specialists.

Juicing and Juice Supplements   Freshly prepared carrot juice, which contains Beta-carotene which, with the help of the liver, breaks down enzymes into Vitamin A analog (abscisic acid). Abscisic acid (CIS 14) and mycelized Vitamin A (100,000 IU/day for 30 days) added to the carrot juice helps to stimulate the immune system.

Daily Nutrient Supplement Blend Patients are encouraged to take a daily blend of Antioxidants, Vitamins, B Complex, Minerals, Trace Elements and Phyto-nutrients which the Center has formulated for improved health and maximum enhancement of the immune system.

Detoxification Cleansing of the colon to remove undesirable flora and bacterial toxins, couple with the subsequent addition of fiber, acidophilus and bifidus to the diet is very important in promoting a healthy, functional digestive system.

With care and attention, it is possible to create and follow a diet which will not detract from but will significantly enhance the body's ability to fight disease. A series of such diets has been carefully developed at the LFMC. During two days of each week the staff nutritionist holds group classes for Center patients and their attending family members to provide specific nutritional instruction for both new and recovering patients. An excellent cookbook written by Ana Canales is devoted to menus and recipes that enhance and strengthen the immune system. An abridged version of <u>The Cookbook</u> appears as an appendix to this book.

One of the more difficult tasks for patients upon returning home is to maintain compliance with the nutritional and clinical programs. Knowing this the staff takes an active support role by calling patients and discussing concerns or problems.

THE PSYCHOLOGICAL SUPPORT PROGRAM

"Stress can make you sick. People say they get sick from overwork or a hectic lifestyle, and they're not far from the truth—the relationship between stress, nutrition and the immune system can have a profound affect on your health." (Dale Ames Kline, M.S., C.N.S.D., Eureka, California).

Years ago Dr. Virginia Livingston realized there are many possible causes for a person's immune system to become depleted, and that emotional and physical stress play huge roles. She was among the first medical researchers to recognize stress and stress-related psychological variables as a possible source of decline for a healthy person's immune system. Her extraordinary insight led her to surmise that emotional support, psychological counseling, group therapy and spirituality would contribute to a positive outlook and thereby enhance the immune system and aid in the process of healing. Hence she incorporated a psychological and emotional component in the Livingston Center's treatment program. The Center has had a psychologist on the staff for over twenty years.

It was not until the mid 1980's that the medical community, spurred by the worldwide AIDS crisis, began to investigate more fully the role the immune system plays in a person's overall health, illnesses and healing. This was a concept well understood by Dr Livingston and one that by this time was already incorporated into her program in San Diego. Today these concepts are generally accepted in the field of medical psychology, in which it is common to discuss the relationship of stress to various illnesses with patients.

Now the formal field of "psychoneuroimmunology" incorporates the clinical research of the past forty years into an understandable and useful tool in preventive medicine and therapeutic programs worldwide. It enhances an individual's ability to recognize and cope with the negative effects of stress and facilitates the natural defenses and immune responses to chronic diseases. Psychoneuroimmunology brings the ancient understanding of the mind-body connection to modern clinical treatment.

Current research generally understands stress not as an outside event, but rather as a particular reaction or response to an event. Thus, most people's experience of stressful states does not necessarily come from highly negative experiences or events in their lives, but rather from a pattern of consistent negative thinking. In this sense, stress is seen as a learned response—a response the patient can chose to avoid. Clinical psychology regards many forms of depression and anxiety problems (which can be considered stressful because of their upsetting and long term effect) to be the result of pessimism and negative cognitions. In these situation the stress response is "optional" and new ways of thinking, perceiving, or evaluating can be learned. On the other hand, there may be times when a series of highly negative events may occur in a person's life. This often happens when a life-threatening disease, such as cancer, is diagnosed. Then, even the most knowledgeable and sophisticated individual, who is accustomed to managing emotional responses, may well experience a period of profound stress.

Regardless of the underlying cause of stress, the impact on an individual's immune system will be damaging. The body's natural life-saving, emergency response, often referred to as the fight-flight response, can become chronic as a result of normal life stresses and can severely depress the immune system. In 1997 Dr. Claude B.

Lambert, M.D. found that an important neurological connection exists between the brain and the immune system. Through this connection, negative stress increases the production of "stress hormones", including the HCG hormone, which, in turn, inhibit the immune system and fuel the growth of the cancer-causing Progenitor cryptocides mycobacteria. Conversely, research has shown that such a chronic automatic stress response can be countered by eliciting the relaxation response. A patient's ability to relax has a significantly positive, direct and measurable effect on the immune system. This includes increases in the immune system's production of white blood cells, natural killer (NK) cells, T-cells, B-cells and Complement, all so essential in fighting and preventing serious, chronic diseases.

To assist in promoting and restoring the function of its patients' immune systems, the LFMC program incorporates psychoeducational classes, individual health counseling and experiential exercises as important elements in its clinical protocol. Most patients believe that stress played some role in contributing to the onset of their illness; therefore, it is important to address these concerns as an essential part of their treatment program. Classes taught by an instructor qualified in the field of psychonuroimmunology are as important a part of the overall Livingston program as the clinical and nutritional components. One of the main goals of the classes is to teach patients that by managing the way they respond to stressful circumstances, they are gaining control over the harmful effects of stress on their bodies—in particular their immune systems. When psychological counseling is desired or indicated, appropriate recommendation for referral is made. Other psychotherapeutic elements of the program are optional and can be tailored to the needs of each patient.

New patients and their families or support persons are given an introduction to the field of psychoneuroimmunology which includes a basic overview of the history of mind-body medicine up to and including current research findings in the field. Stress research has been remarkably consistent over the last forty years. Virtually no studies have indicated that stress may have a positive effect on health or healing. A brief history of research linking psychological variables with health and healing is also discussed. While research results in this area are not as conclusive as those in the area of stress, there are many good studies that show a connection between certain psychological attributes and increased healing rates, better outcomes from surgery and an improved quality of life. These attributes include a positive attitude, emotional support, prayer and spirituality, optimism, a sense of responsibility for one's own health and control of the treatment process. In addition to giving an overview of the research in mind-body medicine, the introductory class also helps set the stage for more practical application of stress management techniques, which patients can apply when they return home.

Conducting group classes allows and encourages mutual support and interaction with others. The class format is both lecture and discussion. In addition to the general principles of stress management, specific topics include dealing with cancer, health care systems, family and relationship difficulties, and work-related stress. Patients have an opportunity to learn new ways of reframing the way they think about their lives and methods of creating more positive and optimistic attitudes, thus lessening the harmful effects of stress.

Patients are also invited to meet individually with the psychologist to discuss their concerns. Occasionally these sessions may focus on such health-related issues as implementing the Livingston program at home, or fears about death and dying. The focus of these sessions is not therapy, or psychological counseling, or even problem solving, but rather helping each patient recognize the impact stress may have on their immune system and on impeding their healing.

Recent research studies have shown stress levels in family members of patients to be virtually the same as those of the patients. Therefore, while the needs of the patient are paramount at the Center, special attention also focuses on the family member, spouse, significant other or friend who accompanies the patient. Family members are encouraged to participate along with the patient in every aspect of the program. Support persons are taught how to give injections, as well as try their hand at vegetarian cooking. In addition, a group meeting called the "Caregivers' Class" is held to help identify and support all the special needs and concerns of those providing care for the patient.

The psychoneuroimmunotherapy program at LFMC has two approaches—physiological and psychological. Physiological stress occurs when the person's fright-flight response is activated, or the person's level of arousal is high and sustained over an extended period of time. Livingston patients are taught to identify and experience their emotions and to distinguish them from the harmful and destructive state of stress. Emotions are a normal and positive experience of life. Positive emotions and even the normal expression of negative emotions are associated with a higher quality of life. However, the effects of holding on to negative emotions will, over time lead to stressful states such as anxiety and depression. These, in turn, will have a profound negative impact on health in general and the immune system in particular. The Livingston program aims at helping patients create more neutral responses to life events and personal circumstances. Understanding that it is almost impossible to adopt a positive attitude at all times, the staff feel it is more reasonable to help patients maintain equilibrium and balance.

The Livingston seminars provide the patient with a variety of techniques which help to elicit the basic, relaxation response and thereby return the body to a baseline condition. These classes normally consist of the following approaches:

1. Relaxation techniques. These include progressive muscle relaxation and autogenic training. The first approach outlines the muscular-skeletal system and teaches the patient to alternatively tense and relax various muscle groups, thereby providing a total release of body tension. The second approach, autogenics, uses the neurological or central nervous system to create a sense of calm and relaxation in the body. Patients are taught to simply allow the tension and stress to dissipate from the body.
2. Meditation. Probably the most researched area in the field of mind-body medicine, meditation has been shown to produce significant changes in physiological functioning. When we create a state in which the brain, or more specifically the cerebral cortex, is quieted, the body

responds by defaulting to a deep state of relaxation. This state is more profound than that produced by the relaxation techniques, and it creates positive changes in both physiological and psychological functioning.

3. Visualization. In a typical visualization, participants are invited to remember a previous experience when they felt safe, comfortable and relaxed. The facilitator supports and encourages patients to involve as many of their senses as they can. Typical sensory impressions may involve memories of warm sunshine, trees or soaring birds. Based on the Simonton research, visualizations also include a specific self-generated set of images. These personal physical or symbolic images are focused on healing and recovery. The sessions are accompanied by recorded music, designed by a music therapist. The tempo begins at about 80 beats per minute and gradually slows to about 60 beats per minute—the optimum number of heartbeats in a totally relaxed state. LFMC patients report that it is easier to relax when this type of music is combined with the

relaxation exercises. Recent research studies show mantra meditation and visualization as very effective methods for inducing the relaxation response and increasing the function of the immune system. And the results can last up to twelve hours!

The goal of the entire psychological program at the Center is to help patients recognize the importance of reducing the damaging effects of stress on their immune system. The number one priority is to facilitate, through the mind-body connection, an avenue to health and healing through improved immunity to disease. The psychological approach utilizes cognitive-behavioral techniques through which patients are taught how their thoughts influence their feelings. The staff discusses numerous examples and gives specific suggestions as to ways to manage personal responses to difficult or demanding situations. Patients are taught ways to control stress levels in their bodies by discovering and learning new ways to think about situations or events in their lives.

SUMMARY

The Livingston Foundation Medical Center's program is composed of three major components. The first is the medical program which emphasizes the use of antigens to enhance the depleted immune system's ability to overcome disease. The second is the use of nutrition and nutritional supplements to further strengthen the immune system, and the third is psychological support and patient health counseling which teach patients to aid in their own recovery process and to sustain good health after they leave the program.

Dr. Virginia Livingston was a physician with great vision. Well before conventional medicine recognized the possibility of environmental factors as a cause of cancer, she discovered the Progenitor cryptocides mycobacterium and its connection to the growth of cancer cells. Well before conventional medicine recognized the importance of the mind-body connection in the healing process, she had incorporated those concepts in her treatment program. Well before conventional medicine recognized the importance of a healthy immune system in the fight against chronic, debilitating and fatal diseases, she had developed a program to nurture and strengthen this miraculous system. Today, thanks to the vision of her family, patients at the Livingston Foundation Medical Center in San Diego, California continue to reap the benefits of the life work of this remarkable woman.

APPENDIX <u>THE COOKBOOK</u>

INTRODUCTION

In 1949, almost fifty years ago, Dr. Virginia Livingston isolated a microorganism that she believed to be a cancer-causing agent. Like many medical and scientific discoveries, this one came about by accident. But when she went on to experiment with laboratory animals, inoculating them with the organism, they developed cancer; further, identical acid-fast microbes in tumors she collected from nearby hospitals, when cultivated and injected into laboratory animals, led to evidence of cancer cells.

Dr. Livingston, and her colleagues at the New York Academy of Sciences gave the organism its bacteriological classification, <u>Progenitor Cyptocides</u> (we refer to it as the PC microbe). And Dr. Virginia devoted the rest of her life to investigating the characteristics of the PC microbe. These investigations, in New York and in Southern California, convinced her that the correct diet plays an invaluable part in building a strong, disease-resistant immune system.

At the Livingston Foundation Medical Center, the immune-boosting diet developed by Dr. Virginia is a major component in our treatment of immunodeficiency diseases. We—and, to be sure, others—continue to investigate the changing world of good health and to advocate nutrition-based resistance to disease.

In continuing Dr. Virginia's work, and through supportive and caring relationships with our patients at the Center, we have come to realize that a healthy, nutritious, immune-boosting diet requires some effort to achieve. It requires, in more or less equal parts, some research and understanding, some sacrifice, some extra effort, some discretionary shopping practices, some shedding of old habits and acquiring of new ones—that is, a general readjustment of our nutritional lifestyle.

Generally speaking, foods bought from the supermarket shelves of America today—fruits and vegetables, for the most part—do not have the same vitamin and mineral strength as they did when they sprouted from the ground or were picked from the tree.

Dr. Virginia often cited Emanuel Cheraskin, M.D., D.D.S., of the University of Alabama School of Medicine, whose thesis was that "from the garden to the gullet", the food on your table has lost at least half of its nutrients. This is because the mineral content of most America's arable soil has been reduced, most notably by pesticides and chemicals (10 percent), and because foods must be transported great distances today for consumption (10 percent). In fact, one study showed that a carrot eaten by an American today has far fewer nutrients in it than a carrot eaten by his Third World counterpart, simply because the latter probably got the carrot less than a mile from his home, whereas the more affluent American had his shipped from hundreds, even thousands, of miles away.

Dr. Cheraskin's analysis now leaves us with 80 percent. Storage in warehouses and supermarket shelves robs another 10 percent of nutrients, and freezing or premature harvesting takes another 10 percent. Washing and scrubbing in preparation for cooking, 5 percent. Now consider the way most Americans prepare their food, by boiling, broiling, baking, and frying. Broccoli and spinach, for example, are usually boiled to death, removing 50 percent of the nutrients in these potentially strong immunity-boosting vegetables. Meat gets overcooked, potatoes boiled to mush—now you have about 40 percent of the original nutrients on your plate. After considering preservatives (to keep those bugs off the fruit), additives (to make those beets redder), processing (cheese), sweeteners (like the sugar added to catsup), and on and on, your plateful of dinner may be only at 30 percent of the nutritional power Nature intended for it.

We at the Livingston Foundation believe only a nutritionally informed person can hope to avoid the dietary pitfalls of daily life. In our present society we have the knowledge and skill to avoid or minimize the damages from immunodeficiency diseases with nutritionally powerful diets. There are simple things provided by Nature that we can use to prevent disease, alleviate ill health and prolong life. These "simple things" are our life habits, which include avoiding noxious substances such as alcohol and tobacco and working to avoid or control stress in our lives. Most importantly, we can become educated in the simple principles of good nutrition. In a society commercially oriented to the mass production of cheap food, preservatives to prolong shelf life, exploitation of taste over quality, convenience, attractive packaging, and the hustle-bustle of everyday working life, the trusting and unsuspecting individual can become lost in a jungle of incomprehension, leading to poor health and general deterioration.

When faced with life-threatening disease such as cancer, most people are willing to comply with any program that might prolong life. We have all long known the value of Vitamin C in preventing scurvy and of the B vitamins in fighting pellagra. In the few years since Dr. Virginia's death, in 1990, new evidence has shown betacarotene has disease resistant characteristics. How many of us know what other factors can increase the restorative functions of the body when faced with serious disease?

At the Medical Center we have made certain recommendations to the patient with chronic debilitating diseases such as arthritis, cancer, or any other disabling collagen disease. In particular, we constantly strive to increase the immune potential of the cancer patient through research on nutrition. Based largely on Dr. Virginia's rather stringent original "anti-cancer diet," but modified over the years to accommodate the average person's lifestyle, we have developed a basic food guideline for all of us, healthy or ill, who desire stronger immunity-boosting benefits from their diets.

The guideline has certain outright prohibitions, such as the avoidance of cancer-infected food, refined flour, white sugar, and empty calories devoid of vitamins and minerals. In their place, we have prescribed food rich in minerals and vitamins and high in healing, nutritive substances. We have tried to present food that is palatable; adapted to the digestive capabilities of the sick; readily available; inexpensive; and easy to prepare.

This diet regimen is not intended as a treatment for cancer. It is intended to raise immunity and increase the resistance of the patient to disease.

In addition to providing supplemental vitamins and minerals, we present a natural source of protective foodstuffs. We know that: Vitamin A guards against chemical carcinogenesis; Vitamin C promotes healing; nicotinamide, B12, and riboflavin increase cellular oxidation; and abscisic acid, an analog of Vitamin A, neutralizes human choriogonadotropin (HCG), a hormone that Dr. Virginia found promotes the growth of cancer cells.

Abscisic acid, a little known derivative of Vitamin A, is a key component of the Livingston Foundation Diet. Almost a half century ago, Dr. Virginia determined that the abscisic acid component of Vitamin A appeared to neutralize HCG. The actual chemical reaction is highly complex, but abscisic acid's importance to the immune system is the reason foods highly concentrated in Vitamin A are frequently emphasized in this cookbook.

Finally, a short word about vegetarianism and the general proscription against meat in these recipes.

Vegetarianism has been defined as either "scientific" (or "medical") vegetarianism or "emotional" vegetarianism. Emotional vegetarians are offended by the killing of animals by human beings, or their treatment while alive, or the idea of "predigested" flesh. These vegetarians often state that they won't eat anything "that has a mother", or that "has a face." Their passion is very real.

Dr. Virginia advocated "scientific" vegetarianism, that is, the eating of the healthiest food one can find, and eschewing all food, including meat, that is known to be infected by one substance or another, and which therefore likely harbors the PC microbe in its tissues.

Her early scientific work in the discovery of the PC microbe, her later medical work at Rutgers in New Jersey, and at her clinic in San Diego, California, overshadowed Dr. Virginia's deserved place as a pioneer in the nutrition movement in this country. While Adele Davis, et al., were calling attention to the benefits of vegetarianism (and being ridiculed for it by the meat industry and many other special interests), Dr. Virginia was quietly advocating the avoidance of what she called "contaminated" foods. One of these foods was chicken, which had been found almost universally to be infected with the PC microbe.

The basis of Dr. Virginia's recommendations against meat was not so much the meat, *per se*, as what happens to it on the way to your table. Just as with the "garden to the gullet" deterioration of fruits and vegetables, most meat has been largely "denatured" by the time it reaches your dinner plate. The unhealthy conditions of raising cattle, including the fertilizers and pesticides in their food, contribute in a major way to creating herds of unhealthy animals. Steroids are used to hasten their rate of growth. Many nutritionists believe that children are maturing faster these days—such as earlier onset of menses—because of the steroids in their diets.

Butchering techniques may not be properly selective, so that sick animals are often processed along with the healthy ones. While visible tumors are removed, animals remain systemically infected, and they are thrown into the process. The mass processing of cattle is simply too fast these days to adequately filter out unhealthy animals. Dr. Virginia believed that when *part* of a body is sick, such as a tumor or other organic infection, the *whole* body is sick. Hence, the whole animal should be removed from the process, not just the animal's tumor or infected part.

In many cases, when a patient cannot tolerate a strictly vegetarian diet, modifications can be made to include "cleaner" meat, such as lamb, wild game and fish. These foods have been found to have low incidences of PC microbe infection.

The bottom line is whether one wants to play it safe or gamble: to select the healthiest foods available, or take a chance on foods that have a high probability of contamination. The foods you select should always be of the highest quality.

Everyone, whether well or sick, should have a practical, working knowledge of modern nutrition; and each of us must learn *how* to choose the foods necessary for good health. Dr. Virginia Livingston often quoted this from Thomas Parran, M.D., a former head of the U.S. Public Health Service: "We must all remember that no one becomes well-nourished by accident."

We offer you this guide, with the wish it will help you - (and perhaps your family) - to find good nutrition and good health.

The Cookbook is not presented as a substitute for good medical care, rather as an adjunct to recovery from serious illness that is life-threatening. Many of the principles in this book can be used to great advantage to promote the continuation of good health and to prevent physical degeneration.

DIET: THE KEY TO HEALTH

...and the key to a healthy diet is *balance*. Diets restricted to a preponderance of one kind of food can be dangerous because they are not well-balanced. Both the mind and the body require a *variety* of foods to maintain health. We know that missing nutrients in the diet can lead to disease. What we sometimes don't appreciate is that foods provide many of the same nutrients.

Foods can be categorized according to their nutrient similarities such as grains, vegetables, fruits, beans, nuts and seeds, etc. Although there are major similar nutrients among these groups, there are, however, varying differences among their micro-nutrients. Therefore, the goal is to eat a variety of foods within each group in order to assimilate more of the nutrients required by the body.

Foods vary in their concentration of fats, carbohydrates, and protein, with many foods predominant in one or the other. These foods should be taken in proper proportions, because it is important to closely watch our caloric intake. Fat, for example, is the most concentrated in calories, yielding 9 calories per gram. However, carbohydrates and protein yield only 4 calories per gram. Therefore, foods that have a high concentration of fat should be consumed in moderate amounts, focusing on plant oils such as olive or flax seed. Eating fats and oils in as close to their natural state as possible is very important. Subjecting them to processing and high tempature can lead to carcinogenic molecular changes and the formation of free radicals. This can lead to an increased risk of disease.

Carbohydrates should be consumed in adequate amounts to provide the body with a source of available energy. The majority of plant-based foods are rich in complex carbohydrates, balanced with fiber. Refining these carbohydrates can lead to insulin resistance and obesity—two serious health concerns afflicting our nation's sedentary population. Regulating the type and amount of carbohydrate to the individual's need is essential in maintaining a balance diet.

Your body needs protein for structure and rebuilding of tissues, including muscle, which is constantly being broken down and rebuilt. Protein is derived from a variety of "building blocks" called amino acids. An adult's requirement for protein is only moderate, because an excess will not be utilized, but rather converted into carbohydrates or stored in the body as fat.

In addition, a good exercise regimen is recommended to maintain the delicate balance among these three food elements.

It would be nearly impossible to go to the store and buy a pound of carbohydrates, or a pint of fat, or a package of protein. You must get them in varying degrees from the food you eat. And since all foods contain little "bundles" of fat, carbohydrates, protein, vitamins, minerals, fiber, and water, the proper proportions of these components becomes very important if the body is to digest and utilize micronutrients in perfect balance.

It's been shown that, when components of these complete bundles are isolated, removed and concentrated (such as fat and sugar), then ingested, the body's balance is disturbed. This is because the body cannot efficiently process one component without the presence of others in specific proportions. When it is forced to try, the result is stress to both mind and body—and ongoing stress leads to disease.

Ideally then, foods should be consumed in their complete bundles of components to help bring about and insure ongoing health. For example, vegetables, whole grains, beans and legumes, fruits, nuts, and seeds are completely "bundled" foods. The body can assimilate the micro-nutrients in these foods quite nicely. That is why these food groups are the main constituents in a strict and balanced vegetarian diet.

The following illustration shows these food groups proportionately stacked in a pyramid-type scheme for optimum balance, according to their composition of fat, carbohydrates and protein. Note that the base (or largest percentage of the pyramid) is devoted to carbohydrate-rich foods; the mid-section includes foods with a slightly higher proportion of fat (such as fruits and nuts and seeds), as well as the more refined soy products derived from the whole soybean; and the top of the pyramid contains the high-fat foods (the smallest percentage of the pyramid). In summary, as long as you eat a variety of foods in the proper proportion, it is easy to maintain a balanced vegetarian diet promoting optimum health **The Cookbook** is your guideline to those proper proportions.

**OILS
CREAM
BUTTER
DRESSINGS**

**FRUIT
SOY PRODUCTS
RAW NUTS & SEEDS**

**VEGETABLES

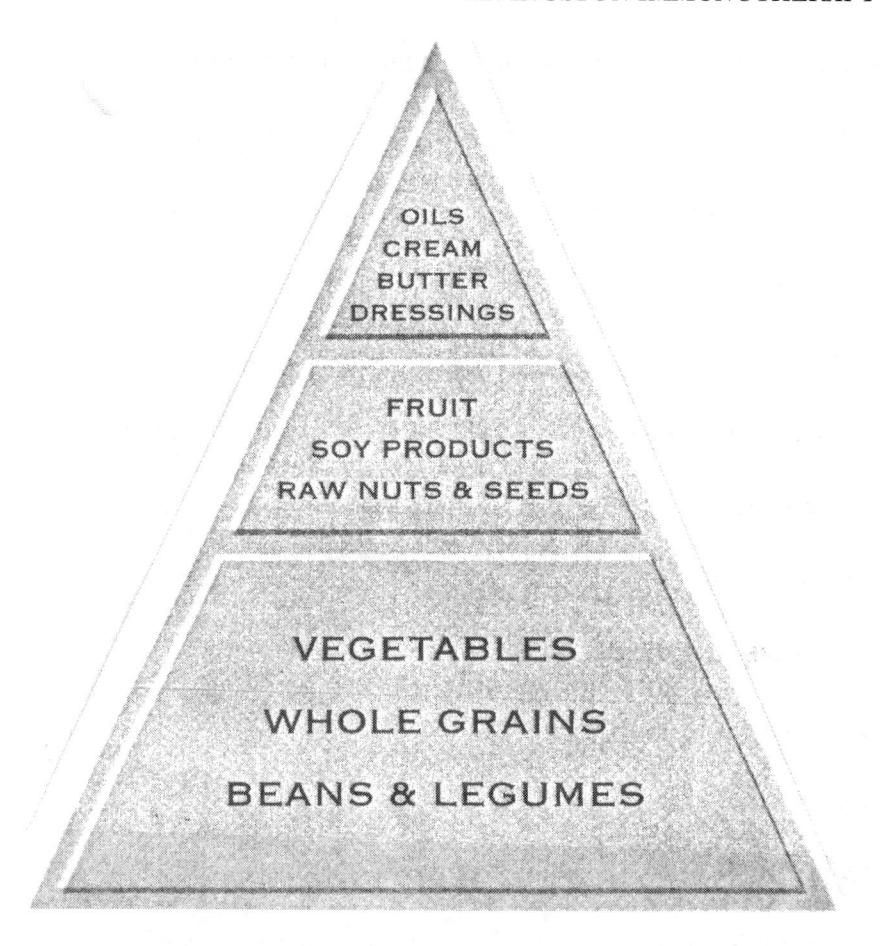

WHOLE GRAINS

BEANS & LEGUMES**

Here are some of Dr. Virginia's prescriptions for healthy eating gleaned from her lifetime of dealing with immune deficiency diseases.

1. Very ill people should consume large amounts of fresh juices and homemade soups. These tend to saturate the system with organically-combined minerals, vitamins and

liver-oxidizing enzymes, which in turn detoxify the body. The exception to this suggestion is when nothing can be kept in the stomach except water, then grain waters are recommended.

2. Eat organically-grown, unsprayed and unfumigated fruits and vegetables when available, or grow them yourself. The soil is a great metabolizer. A home garden - replete with compost, earth worms and natural fertilizers—is an ideal hobby for your dietary lifestyle. Conversely, wilted, pale, flabby, soft-spotted imperfect fruits and vegetables rob you of vitality and immune-building nutrients.

3. Increase your intake of high-potassium foods, such as greens, potatoes, lima beans, nuts and most fruits and vegetables. Try to combine legumes, grains, and leafy vegetables in planning your individual meals.

4. Decrease the high-sodium foods, such as celery and processed salted foods.

5. Learn to substitute:
    - arrowroot for thickening

- yeast or egg replacer for leavening instead of eggs
- oil and butter for shortenings
- soy milk or whipping cream for milk
- low-sodium baking powder, kelp, vegetable herb seasoning or sea salt for iodized salt

6. Add nuts to any recipe to increase the protein content
7. Limit yourself to one or two pieces of citrus fruit per day and eat them whole, except for the skin
8. Carry around a "snack bag" of carrot sticks, broccoli and other raw vegetables, nuts and dried foods.
9. Avoid refined or processed foods, because they are usually robbed of their nutrients. The less refined and more primitive the food stuff, the better.
10. Do not use any milk products, except cream and butter in moderate amounts. Products such as milk, cheese or yogurt contain the hormone prolactin, which stimulates unhealthy cell growth.
11. Bottled water is recommended for drinking and cooking because most municipal water is fluoridated at the plant

before it's even transported to your kitchen. Fluorine is a cumulative enzyme poison which is concentrated by cooking. Also, other unhealthy micro-organisms are often present in tap water.

12. Food should be cooked in stainless steel cookware, iron stone steamers or stainless steel steaming baskets. Avoid the use of pressure cookers, microwave ovens, aluminum pots and utensils.

13. Become a label detective. Read ALL labels. It's difficult, but try to avoid artificial colors, flavors, preservatives and sugar substitutes. Watch out for preservatives such as BHT and BHA. Read labels on products used for sweetening to make sure they contain no artificial sweeteners.

14. Alcoholic beverages, even wine, are not good for sick people. The same is true of soft drinks and iced drinks, because they inhibit digestion.

15. Quit smoking and avoid smoke-filled rooms.

16. Get at least eight hours of sleep, plus regular relaxation periods. Exercise daily according to your ability, and if possible, outside.

17. Take hot baths daily to increase circulation. Cultivate a positive mental attitude.

RE-STOCK YOUR PANTRY!

As you read the recipes and comprehend the general tone of *The Cookbook*, you'll begin to alter your shopping habits. Your pantry will take on a totally new look, and these are the foods that should eventually be stocked there.

Beverages Herb teas, sesame or nut milk, soy milk, cereal beverages (eg - Postum), chicory or dandelion teas.

Breads Millet, rye, buckwheat, whole wheat, bran, corn, seven-grain, corn tortillas. Only whole grains - freshly ground and free of preservatives. The abscisins are lost if baked over 300 degrees F.

Cereals Millet, oatmeal, brown and wild rice, buckwheat, alfalfa, groats, barley, cornmeal, oatmeal, cracked wheat and seven-grain. Freshly ground rolled flakes or whole grain only.

Desserts Fresh whole fruits, fresh fruit cocktails, natural fruit gelatin, health desserts made of outlined ingredients.

Fat/Oil	Olive oil, avocados, raw butter if possible, flax oil and unrefined coconut butter.
Fish	Fresh and salt water fish, broiled, baked or poached. Avoid shellfish.
Fruits	Fresh fruits, organically grown if possible. Apples, apricots, bananas, berries, cherries, currants, grapes, guava, mangoes, melon, nectarines, papaya, peaches, pineapple, pears, plums, persimmons, tangerines, unsulfured dried fruits - apples, apricots, figs, peaches and prunes. Where possible, eat the seeds or kernels with the fruit.
Juices	Only freshly pressed juices and frozen pineapple juice. Select from list of fruits and vegetables. Apples and carrot are the most popular. Also, include beet leaves, chicory, escarole, Swiss chard, watercress beets and cucumbers.
Meat	Lamb and its internal organs such as lamb heart and extra fresh lamb liver.

Milk	Substitute soy milk, seed and nut milks such as sesame, sunflower, almond and cashew.
Nuts	Fresh, raw nuts, particularly walnuts, almonds, cashews, pecans and apricot pits. Raw nut butters freshly made in the blender or juicer.
Salads	Use raw fruits and mature vegetables (listed here) shredded or chopped, separate or combined, such as shredded apple and carrot.
Seasonings	Chives, garlic, parsley. Herbs: laurel, marjoram, sage, thyme, savory, kelp, vegetable and herb seasonings without table (sodium) salt.
Seeds	Sunflower, flax, sesame and pumpkin - fresh and raw.
Soups	Homemade soups from listed ingredients; barley, brown rice or millet can be added.
Sprouts	Sprouts to the age of seven days are permitted since Vitamin A and the abscisins are very rich in these; but after eight days, the gibberellins are produced, which promote the rapid growth of seedlings and tumors and neutralize the abscisic acid.

Vegetables Organically grown raw or freshly cooked: Artichokes, asparagus, beets, broccoli, carrots, cauliflower, chives, corn, endive, green and wax beans, kale, legumes, potatoes, spinach, squash, Swiss chard, watercress, and any seasonal vegetable.

FOODS TO AVOID

Naturally, there is a long list of proscribed foods, which are either nutritionally deficient, or cancer-infected, according to Dr. Virginia's theories about the *P. Cryptocides* organism that causes cancer. In any case, these foods are downright bad for you.

Beverages	Alcohol, cocoa, coffee, milk and soft drinks.
Bread	White and blended breads made from white flour.
Cereals	Processed cereals, puffed or sugared. No white rice.
Cheese	Only as directed when recovered.
Desserts	Canned or frozen fruits. All pastries, gelatin, custards, sauces, ice cream, candy, except those made from suggested health ingredients.
Fats/Oils	Shortening, margarine, saturated oils & fats; rancid or continuously heated oils.
Fish	Smoked or salted fish. Fish preserved in antibiotics. **No shellfish.**

Meats	No poultry. No pork in any form including bacon, ham or ribs. No fried, smoked, salted or processed meats such as sausage or cold cuts. **No beef or veal.**
Milk	Only whipped cream and raw butter may be used in moderation.
Nuts	Salted nuts.
Potatoes	Commercial French fries or potato chips.
Soups	Canned or frozen soups, fat stock, bouillion or dehydrated consomme.
Sprouts	Mature sprouts.
Sweets	White refined sugar and sugar products such as candy; all sugar substitutes; honey, except as directed.
Vegetables	Sprayed and canned. Sulfur and high sodium foods. Frozen vegetables preferred to canned when fresh are not available.

VITAMINS

The lively debate about the value of vitamins continues to rage throughout the scientific community. We know that some vitamins have value in preventing deficiency diseases like scurvy (Vitamin C) and rickets (Vitamin D), but only recently have some scientists admitted that vitamins may play a role in promoting optimum health and vitality. Regardless, it seems that with every new study, the medical community as a whole comes a tiny step closer to subscribing to the value of vitamins.

Dr. Virginia believed passionately in the immune-boosting value of some vitamins, the cancer-fighting value of others, and the optimum health value of still others. In fact, her multimodal immunotherapy treatment of cancer patients included large daily doses of specific vitamins. In particular, she believed in the cancer-fighting value of abscisic acid, an analog of Vitamin A, and in the immune-boosting value of Vitamin C, or ascorbic acid.

Readers of this book are encouraged to research for themselves the very latest scientific findings that corroborate many of Dr. Virginia's contentions. Here is a compact reference guide.

VITAMIN A

Vitamin A or retinol, a fat-soluble vitamin, has a special relationship to the epithelial tissues of the body including the skin, eyes, and the mucous membranes lining most of the organs of the body. It has a direct role in vision and is present in a pigment in the retina of the eye. Deficiency tends to create a rough and scaly skin, lack of saliva, easy tooth decay with defective enamel. A deficiency may also produce a dry cough or hoarseness, and a tendency to colds. Vitamin A deficiency may also cause muscular degeneration including the heart. Vitamin A malnutrition of the eyes impairs night vision and also makes daylight vision more difficult. Because of its relationship to the lining cells of the body, lack of it often causes inflammation of the delicate membranes which line the eyelids and cover the eyeball. Very often sores in the mouth, digestive system upsets, urinary tract difficulties, glandular problems, and decreased stomach acid may all be traced to Vitamin A deficiency. There is a good supply of this vitamin in fruits, vegetables (especially the green and yellow ones), nuts, seeds, and fish liver oils. An excess of Vitamin A may be toxic, but cases of toxicosis are rare; Vitamin toxicity can cause falling hair, nausea, and headaches. More often, however, and of far greater concern, is its deficiency.

VITAMIN A AND ABSCISIC ACID

Recent research has shown that Vitamin A is very protective against carcinogens, and lends credence to Dr. Virginia's theory that Vitamin A, which includes abscisic acid among its analogs can protect against cancer. The group of Vitamin A analogs are classified as retinoids, of which abscisic acid, a plant dormin, is a member. Abscisic acid appears to decrease the secretion of choriogonadatropic hormone (CGH) which is present in large amounts in tumor cells. Abscisic acid is present in seeds, nuts, grains, root vegetables, and mature leaves of plants and vegetables, but it decreases rapidly when seeds and nuts are soaked. It is also destroyed by heating to 250 degrees.

VITAMIN B1 (THIAMIN)

Vitamin B1 is valuable in the metabolism of carbohydrates and necessary for proper nerve function. Vitamin B1 deficiency can cause neuritis, irritability, insomnia, loss of appetite, abnormal heart action, poor circulation, enlarged heart, constipation and gas formation. Ordinary cooking does not destroy this vitamin, but adding soda to vegetables to make them look fresh does destroy Vitamin B1, as well as many others. Other indications of a deficiency of Vitamin B1 are nausea, vomiting, loss of appetite, headaches, general weakness, muscle cramps, sensation of burning in the feet, ear noises, difficult breathing. The richest sources available of Vitamin B1 are wheat germ, virgin yeast, whole wheat, peas and nuts.

VITAMIN B2 (RIBOFLAVIN)

Vitamin B2 is an important factor for growth and development. It is not stored in the body and is affected by light but not by air or heat. It helps to convert starches and sugars into energy. Often the first sign of deficiency is dimness of vision at a distance or in poor light. Other signs of deficiency are poor appetite, abdominal cramps, weight loss, dark red tongue, cracks in corners of the mouth, a pale, anemic appearance, and premature aging. This vitamin is not destroyed by heat but is destroyed by alkaline solutions, by addition of soda while cooking, or when exposed to strong light. Persons lacking this vitamin become sensitive to strong light. Good sources of this vitamin are green leafy vegetables, especially the outer leaves, which contain *five times* as much Vitamin B2 as the inner leaves. Other sources are beets, nuts, fruits, whole wheat bread, and fish.

NIACIN AND NIACINAMIDE

Niacin is one of the most important vitamins in alleviating schizophrenia and autism. This vitamin comes in two chemical forms, niacin and niacinamide. These have been extremely useful in treating moodiness, disorientation, lack of ability to concentrate, anxiety and irritability. Niacin often causes a flushing or tingling in the neck, forearms and hands soon after taking the vitamin but lasts only a few moments. However, non-flush tablets are just beginning to be manufactured. Niacinamide and niacin aid circulation and cell metabolism. The other B vitamins and Vitamin C need to be present for niacin to be effective.

VITAMIN B6 (PYRIDOXINE)

Vitamin B6 has a soothing or sedative effect on the nerves. It is an important factor in preventing tooth decay. In animal experiments it has been learned that pyridoxine is necessary for proper functioning of the pancreas, especially in the insulin producing cells. Deficiency of this vitamin may result in oily skin, dizziness, nausea, fatigue, restlessness, stiffness of leg, trembling of limbs, a shuffling walk, and even anemia. The body needs magnesium to metabolize this vitamin. A form of iron-deficiency anemia can be brought on by inadequate amounts of Vitamin B6. Sources of this vitamin are available in corn oil, virgin yeast, honey, cabbage, whole grains, bread and fish.

VITAMIN B12 (CYANOCOBALAMIN)

Vitamin B12 is vital for blood-forming organs of the bone marrow, and is needed in the formation of hemoglobin. Cobalt and Zinc are necessary for the body to produce it. Although it is absolutely necessary to make healthy blood, it takes only very small amounts to accomplish its function. Results of a deficiency can cause pernicious anemia. Other symptoms of deficiency are lack of nerve reflexes, a shuffling gait, loss of sense of the position of the feet. Insufficiency decreases production of sex hormones, retards development of the breasts, ovaries and other sex organs. In other words, females become less feminine and males less masculine. Sources of this vitamin are eggs, salt water fish, virgin yeast, wheat germ and soybeans. Meat contains more of this vitamin, hence vegetarians must insure an adequate supply, preferably by addition to their usual food intake.

VITAMIN C

Vitamin C is important in the synthesis of intercellular cement, or collagen, which supports and aids in the nourishment of every cell. The strengthening of collagen, as well as other supportive tissues of the body prevents the spread of bacteria, viruses, and other infectious elements from one cell to another, keeping them from penetrating the cell. It is in this sense that Vitamin C is considered a strong immune-boosting nutrient. While a healthy adult may need no more than 500 to 1,000 mg. Daily, the amount to protect against disease, and especially its spread, can be many times greater. Some revered scientists recommend 1,000 mg. hourly for some diseased conditions. Biochemists Irwin Stone, Ph.D., and Linus Pauling, a Nobel laureate, believe a *healthy* adult needs at least 5,000 mg. per day. Deficiency may cause bleeding gums, easy bruising, susceptibility to all kinds of infections. In severe cases of deficiency, scurvy occurs, as well as marked loss of energy, pain in the limbs and joints, loosening of teeth and easy bleeding. Vitamin C is high in ripe citrus fruits, but is also present in many fresh vegetables. There is often not enough in one's diet to supply the amounts needed for prevention of diseases such as the common cold. Take ascorbic acid to bowel tolerance in order to determine the level best for you—i.e., when your bowels begin to loosen, scale back your dosage until you reach a comfortable level.

VITAMIN D

Vitamin D promotes bone and tooth development and regulates the absorption and fixation of calcium and phosphorus. It is not affected by heat or oxidation. It is synthesized in the skin by activity of ultraviolet light. Vitamin D is a factor in tissue cell respiration and is essential to maintain a normal basal metabolism. A deficiency of this vitamin produces rickets but can also cause restlessness, general soreness of the muscles, enlargement of liver and spleen, and many diseases caused by softening of bones both in infancy and in the aged. Its main source is fish oils. 2,500 to 5,000 International Units are considered to be the average amount needed daily. It is difficult to overdose when natural oils are used.

VITAMIN E (TOCOPHEROL)

There are actually five forms of Vitamin E, comprising a complex group, but they all act together as one vitamin. This vitamin is needed to maintain normal membranes of red blood cells. It is considered vital for the proper development and functioning of the reproductive organs, and its absence can cause sterility. It supplies oxygen to cells. Much has been written about Vitamin E and its value in preventing arteriosclerosis and heart disease. It accelerates healing of body tissues that have been infected or injured. Its tissue building power is authenticated. Bed sores or pressure sores that will not respond to any other methods, heal rapidly with the use of Vitamin E. Food sources are various plant oils. Its presence in smaller amounts is found in lettuce, brown rice, whole grain cereals, green vegetables, nuts and legumes.

VITAMIN F

Vitamin F consists of the unsaturated fatty acids. These fatty acids offer the most concentrated form of energy to the body. Unsaturated fatty acids combine with phosphorus to form a part of every cell and are particularly concentrated in nerve and brain tissues. These acids prevent high cholesterol build-up in the arteries. Some of the symptoms of lack of unsaturated fatty acids include emaciation, severe skin rashes, kidney disorders, difficulty in healing of even small wounds, interference with the ability to reproduce and shortening of the life span. Good sources of this vitamin are present in all oils, cream, nuts and avocados.

VITAMIN K

Vitamin K is essential for adequate blood clotting to prevent hemorrhages from even small cuts or wounds. Other symptoms can be dark urine, loss of appetite, general itching, slow pulse, and even jaundice. It is an excellent preventive of the tendency to bleeding caused by aspirin. Leafy vegetables are the most common source of this vitamin. It is also synthesized in the intestines by certain bacteria. It is present in fats, oats, wheat, rye, and alfalfa.

VITAMIN P (BIOFLAVINOIDS)

Vitamin P, also known as citron, is similar to Vitamin C in its general action. While whole Vitamin C acts mainly on the intercellular cement that binds cells together, Vitamin P has its main effect in strengthening the walls of the capillaries, thus preventing tissue fluids from seeping through into the surrounding cells. The interesting reason for the selection of the letter "P" to designate this vitamin was the word "permeable." It was discovered that this substance stabilizes the permeability of blood vessels. The main food source of this vitamin is natural vegetable juices and whole lemon.

CHOLINE

This is one of the B-complex vitamins. It is essential for proper functioning of the liver. *Chole* is the Greek word for "bile," which explains its name. Although synthesized in the body, it is not made in sufficient amounts to meet the need of man. It must therefore be supplied in food. It is essential for growth and for the prevention of fatty livers. It aids in the normal functioning of nerves and the synthesis of some proteins. Results of deficiency may be fatty liver, poor growth, edema, impaired cardio-vascular system, and hemorrhagic conditions in the kidney, heart muscle and adrenal glands. It is found in whole grains, legumes, wheat germ, and in small amounts in vegetables, but most other foods (except flesh foods) have little or no choline.

PANTOTHENIC ACID

Pantothenic Acid is needed for the proper functioning of the entire digestive system, especially the adrenal glands, and is essential for growth. Food processing has removed this vitamin from most food products on the store shelves. There is good reason to believe that a deficiency of this vitamin is a factor in promoting arthritis, gray hair, skin diseases, granulation of the eyelids, digestive disorders and mental depression. Children born of a mother deficient in Pantothenic Acid may be seriously deformed or mentally retarded. This substance is found in royal jelly honey, human milk, wheat bran, virgin yeast, broccoli, molasses, peanuts, and nearly all vegetables.

NOTE

This very brief summary of the role of vitamins in diet is intended only as an incentive to study in depth the elements essential for life in our daily food. The reader is also encouraged to study the role of minerals in the diet, although there are excellent multiple mineral supplements available that will complement the recipes in this book.

BEVERAGES

Juices, Herb Teas, Grain Waters, Nut and Seed Milks

Dr. Livingston always said, *"The very ill need juices primarily."* This is because when you drink vegetable juice, you are consuming many times the concentration of that vegetable than you ordinarily would with a conventional diet; hence, many more micronutrients per unit volume ingested. In other words, to get the nutrients from drinking a few ounces of, say, spinach juice, you would probably have to eat two pounds of spinach.

It is extremely important to buy the best quality of naturally grown produce you can find. It is also imperative that fruits are washed and vegetables scrubbed with a vegetable brush to remove any residual pesticide sprays and harmful toxins that could become concentrated in the juice. It is further recommended that you drink juices as often as you can. Because carrots contain a high concentration of abscisic acid, it is specifically recommended that you drink as much as a quart of carrot juice each day.

Here are some juice combinations for variety of taste:

Equal parts of carrot and apple juice

Equal parts of carrot and cucumber juice

Equal parts of carrot and fresh tomato juice

Equal parts of apple and grape juice (unsweetened)

3 parts of carrot juice to 1 part of spinach juice

3 parts of carrot juice to 1 part cabbage juice

4 parts of carrot juice to 2 parts cucumber juice and 1 part beet juice

All juices should be prepared fresh and consumed within 1 hour of preparation when possible. It is further recommended that a *triturator* type of juicer such as the Champion juicer be used because it efficiently macerates the fruits and vegetables with the least amount of oxidation. Finally, it has been found that grain waters are easily assimilated and digested, and they provide excellent gastrointestinal relief. In all these recipes, a tablespoon of freshly ground whole grain can be added to any juice to neutralize tartness. Always use purified drinking water for teas and grain waters to prevent the taste from being altered by chemicals or minerals found in tap water.

JUICES

Pineapple Carrot Juice

> 1 cup freshly squeezed carrot juice
> 1/2 cup fresh pineapple, cut in cubes
>
> 1. Blend in blender until smooth. Serve immediately.

Mango Splash

> 2 large mangoes, peeled and diced
> 1/2 medium banana
> 1/2 cup cranberry juice
> 1/2 cup orange juice
>
> 1. Blend ingredients together in blender and serve immediately.

Grape Sunset

> 1 cup fresh grape juice
> 1 cup cranberry juice
>
> 1. Mix together and serve immediately.

TEAS & WATERS

Peach Blossom Tea

1 tsp. peach blossoms
1 cup boiling water

1. Steep for 5 minutes and strain.

Lemon Tea

1 tsp. lemon grass tea
1 tsp. lemon balm tea
1 tsp. lemon verbena tea
1 tsp. citrus blossom tea or fresh citrus blossoms such as orange or lemon
1 quart boiling water

Steep for 5 minutes and strain.

Rose Hip Tea

2 tsp. rose hips
2 cups water

1. Bring water to a boil. Add rose hips. Cover and simmer for 15 minutes. Let cool and strain.

Grain Meal Water

1 tbsp. any whole grain or mixture such as rye, rice, barley or millet
2 cups drinking water

1. Grind grain and mix with cold water. Bring to a boil in a sauce pan. Lower heat and simmer for 1 hour. Cool and serve. Do not store for over 5 days.

Barley Water

2 ounces whole barley
3 pints drinking water

1. In a sauce pan, boil barley and water until the water is reduced by half. Strain and cool. Do not store for more than 5 days.

Rice Water

1 tbsp. rice, ground in flour mill
2 cups drinking water

1. In a sauce pan, mix rice with cold water. Bring to boil. Lower heat and cook for 5 minutes stirring constantly. Cool. Do not store for more than 5 days.

MILKS AND CREAMS

Almond Milk

2 cups drinking water
1 cup almonds
1/4 cup apple juice (optional)
1 tsp. sea salt

1. Blend until smooth. Add more water or almonds to adjust to desired consistency. Apple juice sweetens the milk.

Cashew Milk

2 cups drinking water
1 cup cashews
1 tsp. honey OR 1/4 cup apple juice

1. Blend until smooth. Add more water or cashews to adjust to right consistency.

Nut Cream

1 tbsp. raw cashews
1 tbsp. raw almonds
1 tbsp. raw sesame seeds
3/4 cup drinking water
2 tbsp. coconut juice
1/4 tsp. vanilla
1/2 tsp. raw honey

1. Grind nuts and seeds in blender until fine. At high speed add water until combined and blend with other ingredients until smooth. Serve with breakfast cereals or fruit.

BREAKFAST FOODS

Cereals, Pancakes, Muffins and Much More

Breakfast is the most often forgotten meal for most Americans, yet we know that breakfast is crucial to maintaining good health as it is truly the meal in which we "break fast". We should not skip breakfast at all; simple, healthful meals requiring a little time to prepare should always be taken. When time allows, preparation of an expanded meal will always be appreciated by your newly awakened self!

Fruit Nut Granola

    3 cups rolled oats
    1 cup wheat flakes
    1 cup rye flakes
    1 cup bran
    1 cup dried apples, chopped
    1/2 cup dates, chopped
    1/2 cup golden raisins
    1/4 cup diced apricots, chopped
    1/4 cup dried bananas
    1/2 cup cashews, chopped
    1/4 cup sunflower seeds
    1/2 cup raw honey
    1/2 cup hot water
    1 tbsp. pure vanilla extract

1. Combine all dry ingredients, fruits and nuts in a large bowl.
2. In a small mixing bowl, combine honey, hot water and vanilla. Add to dry ingredients and mix thoroughly with hands to coat all ingredients.
3. Spread on a baking sheet, place in a 250° F. oven and bake for 1 hour, stirring every 15 minutes or until golden brown. Let mixture cool completely and store in a sealed container for up to two weeks.

Makes 9 cups.

Creamed Kasha with Seeds and Fruit

1 cup kasha (buckwheat groats)
4 cups water
1 tsp. sea salt
1/2 pint fresh or frozen berries
1/2 cup golden raisins
2 tbsp. raw honey
1 tbsp. lemon or lime juice
1 tsp. pure vanilla extract
1/2 cup sunflower seeds

1. Grind kasha in a blender or coffee mill. In a medium sauce pan, blend kasha with 1 cup water until smooth. Add remaining water and salt.
2. Bring to a simmer, stirring constantly. Cover and simmer for 15 minutes, stirring occasionally. Add more water as necessary.
3. While kasha cooks, puree berries in a blender or food processor. Put pureed berries through a sieve to remove seeds. Add honey, lemon juice and vanilla to taste. Set aside.

4. When kasha has finished cooking, add sunflower seeds and raisins. Serve in individual bowls with berry sauce on the side.

Serves 2

Cashew Oat Waffles

2 cups rolled oats
1/3 cup raw cashews
1/2 tsp. salt
1 tbsp. oil
2 1/4 cups water

1. Combine all ingredients in blender. Blend until light and foamy. Let mixture stand while waffle iron is heating. Blend again briefly, and bake in hot waffle iron for 8 to 10 minutes until nicely browned.

Makes 4 waffles

Apple Cakes

1 cup cornmeal
1/2 cup garbanzo bean flour
1 tsp. cinnamon
1 cup apple juice
1 tbsp. raw honey
cup apple, scrubbed and grated

1. Mix together cornmeal, flour and cinnamon. Add apple juice and honey, stirring well. Fold in grated apples.
2. Spoon batter onto non-stick griddle. Cook for 3-5 minutes over medium heat until bubbles begin to appear. Turn once to brown other side.

Serves 6

Simple Muffins

2 cups whole wheat pastry flour
2 tsp. baking powder (non-aluminum)
1/2 tsp. sea salt
2 cups nut milk
2 tbsp. applesauce
1/2 tsp. vanilla

1. Combine dry ingredients. Combine wet ingredients. Fold together until just moistened. Spoon into lightly oiled or non-stick muffin tins. Bake at 350° for 25-30 minutes.

Makes 12 muffins

Oatmeal Apple Muffins

1 1/2 cups rolled oats
1 cup shredded raw apple
1/4 cup apple juice
1 tsp. fresh lemon zest
1/4 cup safflower oil
1/2 tsp. sea salt
1/2 cup currants
1/4 cup nuts, chopped

1. Combine all ingredients. Let stand for 5 minutes to moisten all ingredients. Mix well.
2. Place in greased muffin cups. Bake at 375° for 25 minutes. Serve with unsalted butter and honey.

Makes 12 muffins

Spinach Omelet

1/4 cup olive oil
1 1/2 cups fresh spinach, chopped
1 1/2 cups swiss chard leaves, chopped
1 clove garlic, peeled and mashed
8 egg replacer, well beaten
1/3 cup soy parmesan cheese
1 tbsp. parsley, finely chopped
1 tbsp. fresh basil, finely chopped
2 tbsp. butter

1. Heat oil in large skillet. Add spinach, chard and garlic. Cook mixture until oil is absorbed and leaves have wilted. Cool slightly. Add eggs, cheese, parsley and basil.
2. Heat butter in omelet pan. Pour in egg mixture. Cook over medium heat for 10-12 minutes to set omelet.

Serves 4

Wild Rice Scramble

2 tbsp. butter
1/4 cup celery, finely chopped
1/4 cup green bell peppers, finely chopped
8 egg replacer
1/3 cup cream
1 cup cooked wild and brown rice
1/2 tsp. salt
1/2 tsp. black pepper

1. Heat butter in a large skillet. Sauté celery and green peppers over medium heat until soft.
2. Lightly beat eggs with cream. Add wild rice. Pour egg mixture over vegetables in skillet. Scramble until eggs are set but still soft. Season with salt and pepper.

Serves 4

Corn Breakfast Cake

TOPPING
1/2 cup unsweetened coconut
1/2 cup raw apple, shredded
1/2 cup pecans, chopped
1/4 cup raw honey
1/4 cup unsalted butter, melted

CAKE
1 cup cornmeal
1 cup soy flour
2 tsp. baking powder (non-aluminum)
1 tsp. cinnamon
1/2 tsp. nutmeg
1/2 tsp. allspice
1/2 tsp. sea salt
2 tbsp. unsalted butter, melted
1 2/3 cup warm water
2 tbsp. raw honey

1. Combine all ingredients for topping in a small bowl. Set aside.
2. Combine dry ingredients. Combine water, butter and honey. Mix together until just moistened. Spoon into lightly oiled round cake pan. Top with fruit mixture. Bake at 375° for 20 minutes.

Serves 6

SANDWICHES

Delicious, whole grain products are currently available in markets everywhere, making it a simple feat to create a delectable sandwich in no time.

Bananarama

   2 slices whole grain bread
   1 tbsp. nut butter (cashew, almond, etc.)
   1 tbsp. apple butter
   1/2 medium banana, sliced lengthwise
   1 oz. sprouts
   1/2 tsp. cinnamon

   1. Toast bread and spread one slice with nut butter and the other with apple butter. Place banana, sprouts and cinnamon on one slice, and top with the other.

Serves 1

Carroty Wich

   2 cups carrots, scrubbed and shredded
   1/4 cup golden raisins, chopped
   1/4 cup cashews, chopped
   1/4 tsp. cinnamon
   2 tbsp. lime juice
   1/2 cup eggless mayonnaise
   4 slices whole grain bread

1. Toss carrots, raisins, cashews, cinnamon and lime juice together. Bind with mayonnaise. Divide carrot mixture and spread onto two slices of bread. Cover with the other two slices.

Serves 2

Tofu Sandwich Spread

32 oz. tofu
1 cup carrots, grated
1/2 cup green onions, sliced with tops
2 tbsp. nutritional yeast
2 tbsp. fresh lemon juice
1 tbsp. soy sauce
1 tbsp. olive oil
2 garlic cloves, crushed
2 tsp. curry powder
2 tsp. ginger powder

1. Drain tofu well. Meanwhile, grate carrots and slice onions. Mash tofu with a fork until crumbly.
2. Mix all ingredients together until well blended. Let stand in refrigerator for at least one hour.

    This spread is great served on a seeded, whole grain bread with a variety of vegetables such as thinly sliced zucchini, cucumbers, tomatoes and lettuce. You might enjoy filling whole wheat pita pockets with tofu spread, sprouts and chopped vegetables.

Makes about 4 cups

Berinjela Eggplant Filling

1 small eggplant, baked until soft, then peeled and chopped
3 green olives, pitted
1 clove garlic
1 tsp. fresh lemon juice

1/2 tsp. sea salt
1/2 tsp. black pepper
1/4 cup roasted red pepper, finely diced
3 tbsp. eggless mayonnaise

1. Blend eggplant with olives, garlic, lemon juice, salt and pepper in food processor until mixture is very smooth.
2. Stir in finely diced red peppers and mayonnaise to bind. Chill for 20 minutes to combine flavors. Serve open faced on toasted bread.

Makes 1 1/2 cups

Bruschetta with Tomatoes

2 large ripe tomatoes
4 slices country bread, thickly sliced
2 garlic cloves, peeled and cut in half
4 tbsp. extra virgin olive oil
1 tsp. sea salt
4 large basil leaves

1. Very lightly roast tomatoes over an outdoor grill or gas burner. Peel, then cut horizontally to remove all seeds. Cut tomato halves into strips.
2. Grill or toast bread. Rub with cut side of garlic and lightly drizzle with olive oil.
3. Place tomato strips on toast, salt lightly with sea salt. Tear basil leaves into pieces and place over tomatoes. Drizzle with remaining olive oil. Serve warm.

Serves 2

Grilled Tofu "Jack"

4 tbsp. butter
4 slices whole grain bread
8 slices tofu "Jack" cheese
4 slices ripe tomato
4 slices ripe avocado
2 scallions, thinly sliced

1. Melt 2 tbsp. of butter in a large skillet. Place 2 slices of bread into skillet. Top with cheese slices, tomatoes, avocados and scallions, then remaining slices of bread.
2. Cook over medium heat until bread is well browned. Add remaining butter to skillet and turn sandwiches. Serve when other side has browned.

Serves 2

Italian Hero

1 long loaf whole wheat sourdough bread
4 tbsp. eggless mayonnaise (optional)
1 large tomato, thinly sliced
2 tbsp. olive oil
1 tbsp. fresh basil, chopped
1 medium zucchini, thinly sliced
1/2 tsp. sea salt
1/2 tsp. freshly ground black pepper
1/2 lb. tofu "Jack" cheese, thinly sliced
1 medium red onion, very thinly sliced
1 medium green pepper, sliced into paper thin rounds
2 tbsp. pepperoncini, chopped

1. Slice loaf in half lengthwise. Spread with mayonnaise, if desired.
2. Divide fillings into halves. Layer with half of the tomatoes, then sprinkle lightly with oil and basil. Next, layer with zucchini, then sprinkle with salt and pepper.

Then layer cheese, followed by onion and green pepper. Sprinkle with pepperoncini.

3. Repeat layers and place top of bread over layered filling. Serves 4

Spinach Calzone

DOUGH
2 tsp. active dry yeast
1 cup warm water
1 1/2 cup whole wheat flour
1/2 cup whole wheat pastry flour
1 tsp. sea salt
2 tbsp. olive oil

FILLING
4 tbsp. olive oil
1/2 cup red onions, thinly sliced
1/2 cup red peppers, diced
1 cup black olives
2 cloves garlic, peeled and mashed
3 cups fresh spinach, stemmed and torn
1 tsp. sea salt
1 tsp. black pepper
2 cups tofu cheese, grated

1. Dissolve yeast in warm water. Mix dry ingredients together. Add yeast mixture and oil to form soft dough. Knead for 10 minutes on lightly floured surface to make a silky dough, adding more flour or water as necessary. Set to rise in a warm place for 1 hour. Punch dough down and allow to rise again for 1/2 hour.
2. Meanwhile, heat 2 tbsp. of olive oil in large skillet. Add onions and red peppers. Cook over medium heat until onions are translucent. Add olives and garlic. Cook 3 minutes more. Add spinach, salt and pepper. Turn heat to

high for 1 minute and cover to barely wilt spinach. Cool mixture. Gently toss with cheese.
3. While dough is rising second time, preheat oven to 450°. Roll dough into 12-14 inch circle. Place on baking sheet or pizza stone. Place spinach mixture on one half of dough. Fold other half over first, then crimp edges making sure to seal completely. Brush top with remaining oil.
4. Bake on lowest rack of oven for 20 minutes or until crust is richly browned. Cool for 5 minutes, then serve.

Serves 2

Hot Pita Splits

1 tbsp. olive oil
1 tsp. thyme
1/4 tsp. sea salt
1/4 tsp. black pepper
2 large whole wheat pita rounds
1 cup tofu cheese, shredded
1/2 cup tomatoes, diced
1/4 cup black olives
1/4 cup red onion, thinly sliced
1/4 cup sunflower seeds

1. Mix together olive oil, thyme, salt and pepper.
2. Split pita rounds horizontally. Layer with tofu cheese followed by tomatoes, olives, and onions. Drizzle with seasoned olive oil. Sprinkle with sunflower seeds.
3. Broil 3-5 minutes until tofu cheese is brown and bubbly.

Serves 2

SALADS AND DRESSINGS

In almost every study of longevity, of cultures with low disease rates, of people in virtually every society (including ours) who never get sick, you'll find a common thread among the factors contributing to the health of the target group—RAW VEGETABLES!!

Green Garden Salad

1 head romaine lettuce, washed and leaves torn
1 cup garbanzo beans, cooked
8 cherry tomatoes, quartered
1 small zucchini, grated
1 small carrot, grated
4 radishes, scrubbed and thinly sliced
1/4 cup raw sunflower seeds
1/2 cup Green Goddess Dressing (following recipe)

Toss vegetables and seeds together. Serve with Green Goddess dressing.
Serves 4

Green Goddess Dressing

3/4 cup eggless mayonnaise or San Pasqual mayonnaise
3/4 cup fresh parsley
1 tbsp. onion, chopped finely clove garlic
1 1/2 tsp. kelp or sea salt

Waldorf Salad

1/2 cup eggless mayonnaise
2 tbsp. lemon juice
1 tsp. hot sweet mustard
2 large red apples, cored and diced
1 cup celery, diced
1 cup seedless grapes, halved
1/2 cup walnuts, lightly toasted
washed and torn

1. In a small bowl, whisk together mayonnaise, lemon juice and mustard. Place apples, celery, grapes and walnuts together in a bowl and toss with dressing. Arrange lettuce leaves on a platter or individual plates. Mound salad on top of lettuce and serve.

Serves 4

Clemente's Potato Salad

2 lbs. white potatoes, scrubbed
3 tbsp. cider vinegar
1 large red bell pepper, seeded and diced
1 bunch green onions with tops, sliced
2 stalks celery, sliced finely
1 1/2 cups eggless mayonnaise
1 tsp. sea salt
1 tsp. black pepper
1 tsp. celery seed
1/8 tsp. paprika

1. Boil potatoes in water until tender when pierced but still firm. Drain, then dice into 1/2 inch cubes. Sprinkle with vinegar.
2. Add red bell pepper, green onions and celery. Fold in mayonnaise, sea salt, pepper, celery seed and paprika.

Serves 6

Easy Three Bean Salad

2 cups kidney beans, cooked
2 cups garbanzo beans, cooked
2 cups black-eyed peas, cooked
1/2 cup fresh peas or frozen petite peas, thawed
1/4 cup fresh parsley, chopped
6 green onions with tops, finely sliced
2 cloves garlic, crushed
1 cup Lemon Dressing (following recipe)

1. Drain beans from their liquids. Rinse lightly.
2. Combine beans with peas, parsley, onions and garlic. Toss gently with dressing. Let stand for at least 2 hours for flavors to blend.

Serves 4

Lemon Dressing

1/3 cup lemon juice
1 clove garlic
1/2 tsp. sea salt
1/2 tsp. black pepper
2/3 cup olive oil

1. Combine lemon juice, garlic, salt and pepper. Slowly drizzle in oil and continue to beat until well emulsified. Makes 1 cup.

Chinese Green Noodle Salad

1 1/2 cups Cashew Nut Dressing (following recipe)
1/2 tsp. ginger, ground or 1 tsp. fresh grated
1 tbsp. toasted sesame oil
1 tsp. hot spicy Chinese mustard (optional)
1 lb. Chinese thin rice noodles, cooked and drained
1/2 lb. broccoli, lightly steamed and cut into bite-sized florets
1/2 lb. asparagus, lightly steamed and cut into bite-sized pieces
1 cup Shitake or other oriental mushrooms, sliced
4 scallions with tops, sliced

1. In a small bowl, whisk together Cashew Nut Dressing with ginger, sesame oil and mustard.
2. In large bowl, toss together Chinese noodles, broccoli, asparagus, mushrooms and scallions. Add dressing, tossing well to coat noodles. Chill for 15 minutes to allow flavors to blend.

Serves 4

Cashew Nut Dressing

1 1/4 cups raw cashews
1 1/4 cups drinking water
1/2 cup safflower or olive oil
1/4 cup lemon juice
2 cloves garlic, peeled
2 tsp. onion powder
1 tbsp. vegesal

1. Place all ingredients in a blender. Blend until smooth and creamy. Makes 3 cups.

7 Layer Fruit Salad

1 pint strawberries, hulled and sliced
4 large peaches, peeled and sliced
1 pint blueberries, washed
2 large bananas, peeled and sliced
2 large oranges, peeled, sectioned and cut into bite-sized pieces
5 tsp. fresh lime juice
6 tbsp. coconut, unsweetened
1 cup whipped cream (following recipe)
1/2 cup granola or toasted nuts

1. Assemble layers in 3 quart, clear glass salad bowl. Begin with strawberries. Sprinkle with 1 tsp. lime juice followed by 1 tbsp. coconut. Continue layering fruit in order given, sprinkling each layer with 1 tsp. lime juice and 1 tbsp. coconut as you go. When all fruit has been layered in dish, top with whipped cream. Chill for 15 minutes.
2. Top with granola or nuts just prior to serving.

Serves 4-6

Whipped Cream

1 cup heavy cream
1 tbsp. honey
1 tsp. vanilla

1. In a chilled mixing bowl, beat cream until thickened to form soft peaks. Add honey and vanilla. Continue beating until stiff peaks form. Do not over beat, as cream turns quickly to butter. Makes 1 cup.

SOUPS

Vegetables, Grains and Fruit

Soup, whether thick and filling or clear and light, should have a place in our everyday cuisine. A bowl of fresh soup can serve as a perfect fall or winter luncheon, or as a light supper during the spring and summer months, each bowlful laden with goodness and nutrition. Avoid canned or prepackaged dehydrated soups which are laden with artificial sweeteners, salt, meat stocks and vegetables that have lost almost all of their nutritional value.

Zuke Soup

    1/2 medium yellow onion, chopped
    2 tbsp. olive oil
    6 cups vegetable stock II (see recipe)
    1 clove garlic, minced
    1/2 tsp. black pepper
    1 lb. spinach, washed and shredded
    2 stalks celery, thinly sliced
    3/4 cup split peas, rinsed
    6 cups zucchini, dried
    1/2 tsp. dried basil
    1 tsp. sea salt
    1/4 cup fresh parsley, chopped

1. In a large pot over medium heat, sauté onion and celery in oil until translucent. Add split peas and 4 cups of stock. Bring to boil, then simmer for 30 minutes over low heat.
2. Add zucchini, remaining 2 cups of stock, garlic, basil, salt and pepper. Continue cooking for 10 minutes. Puree in blender or food processor and return to pot. Add spinach and parsley. Continue to cook for 5 to 7 minutes until spinach is wilted. Adjust seasonings and serve warm.

Serves 6

Quick Minestrone Soup

1/4 cup olive oil
1 large onion, chopped
2 tsp. basil
1/2 tsp. cayenne pepper
1 medium carrot, finely diced
1 cup kidney beans, cooked
4 cups drinking water
1/2 cup mushrooms, sliced
1 large green bell pepper, chopped
3 cloves fresh garlic, chopped
2 tsp. oregano leaves
1 tsp. vegesal
1 cup garbanzo beans, cooked
2 cups crushed tomatoes
1 cup whole grain pasta

1. Heat olive oil in large skillet over medium heat. Add chopped pepper, onion and garlic. Saute until limp but not browned. Add spices and carrot and continue to simmer for 2 minutes. Transfer to a soup pot.
2. Add garbanzo beans, kidney beans, tomatoes and water. Cook over medium heat for 15 minutes to incorporate flavors and soften vegetables.

3. Add dried pasta and mushrooms. Continue cooking for 20 minutes or until pasta is tender. Adjust seasonings.

Serves 4-6

Potato Soup with Tomatoes and Basil

3 large tomatoes
1 tbsp. sea salt
2 cups vegetable broth I (see recipe)
1 large onion, sliced
1 cup cream
2 carrots, thinly sliced
2 tsp. black pepper
4 russet potatoes, diced
1 clove garlic, minced
1/4 cup fresh basil leaves, finely shredded

1. Cut tomatoes in half crosswise to remove seeds, reserve juice and finely chop. Place chopped tomatoes, reserved juice, carrots, salt and pepper in an enameled sauce pan over medium heat. When mixture begins to bubble, lower heat and simmer until carrots are soft. Puree should be dense like a tomato sauce for pasta. Increase heat to boil off liquid. Strain puree to remove tomato skins and chill.
2. Place vegetable broth, potatoes, onion and garlic in a medium sauce pan and simmer 15 to 20 minutes until potatoes are very tender and onion is soft. Puree mixture in a blender. Add cream, season to taste and chill in a tureen. Before serving, swirl tomato puree into potato soup and garnish with basil leaves.

Serves 4

Miso Soup

1/2 cup dry wakame or dulse seaweed
1 cup cabbage, thinly shredded
1 medium carrot, sliced thinly on the diagonal
1 medium yellow onion, sliced thinly
1 lb. spinach, thinly shredded
3 cups drinking water
2 tbsp. olive oil
1 tbsp. miso paste (or to taste)

1. Soak seaweed for 15 minutes in 1 cup of water. Cut into small pieces.
2. Meanwhile, prepare other vegetables. Sauté cabbage, carrot and onion in oil for 5 minutes only.
3. Add remaining 2 cups water and seaweed. Simmer for 20 minutes. Dilute miso with small amount of broth. Stir into soup, mix well and serve.

Serves 4

Cream of Mushroom Soup

1/4 oz. dried porcini mushrooms
2 1/2 cups fresh mushrooms brushed clean with vegetable brush and, chopped
1/4 cup onion, finely chopped
5 cups vegetable stock II (see recipe)
4 tbsp. butter
1/4 cup whole wheat pastry flour
1 cup cream
2 tsp. sea salt
2 tsp. black pepper
1 tbsp. fresh thyme, finely chopped
1/4 cup sauterne or other sweet white wine (optional)

1. In a small bowl, place porcini mushrooms. Pour just enough boiling water over to cover. Let sit 15 minutes to

soften. Strain soaking liquid through a very fine strainer and reserve. Chop mushrooms finely.
2. In a stock pot, bring stock to boil. A fresh mushrooms and onion in stock. Simmer for 20 minutes. Pass vegetables and stock through a sieve. Place back on burner over low constant heat adding procini mushrooms and the reserved liquid.
3. Work butter and flour together to make a paste. Whisk into the gently simmering soup to thicken. Add cream, salt, pepper and fresh thyme. Heat for 5 more minutes. Add wine just prior to serving.

Serves 6

Avocado Tomato Soup

5 large ripe tomatoes, diced
2 large ripe avocados, diced
3 scallions, sliced thinly
1/4 cup almonds, ground
1 cup vegetable broth I (see recipe)
1 tsp. kelp or sea salt
1 lemon, juiced

1. Combine all ingredients. Serve either chilled or heated to just below 115°.

Serves 2-4

Fruit Gazpacho

1/2 cup strawberries, sliced
1 cup grapes, sliced
1/2 cup oranges, sliced with white underpeel intact
1 cup mango, diced
1/2 cup blueberries
1 cup fresh apple juice
1/2 cup fresh orange juice
2 tbsp. lime juice

1/4 tsp. black pepper
12 fresh mint leaves

1. Combine all fruits with juices and pepper in non-corrosive bowl. Chill thoroughly. Serve with fresh mint garnish.

Serves 4

Vegetable Stock I

2 medium leaks, washed and chopped
6 carrots, scrubbed and chopped
1 small bunch of parsley, chopped
2 tsp. dried leaf marjoram
4 medium onions, chopped with skins left on
2 celery ribs with tops, chopped
2 bay leaves
1 tsp. fresh thyme
1-1/2 gallons drinking water

1. Combine all ingredients in large stock pot. Bring to a boil. Reduce heat and simmer 1 hour.
2. Cover a colander or strainer with a double liner of cheesecloth. Strain stock through cheesecloth. Cool completely. Refrigerate or store in freezer to keep longer than two days.

Vegetable Stock II

4 large onions, halved with skins intact
1 bunch celery with tops intact
1-1/2 gallons drinking water
3 bay leaves
6 large carrots, scrubbed
2 tbsp. olive oil
1 bunch parsley stems
1 tbsp. fresh thyme

1. Place onions, carrots and celery in baking pan. Dribble with olive oil and roast in 400 F. oven for 45 minutes until vegetables are well darkened.
2. Transfer vegetables to stock pot. Cover with water. Add parsley stems, bay leaves and thyme. Bring mixture to a boil, then simmer 1 hour.
3. Cover a colander or strainer with a double liner of cheesecloth. Cool completely and refrigerate or store in freezer to keep longer than two days.

PASTA

While the word *pasta* simply indicates the generic form of the multitude of products made from semolina and water. It is the semolina (wheat) that lends both the substance and nutrition to the dish. Be creative with your sauces and accompaniments.

Pasta Fresca

    1 lb. whole wheat spaghetti
    2 garlic cloves, minced
    1/2 cup fresh basil, thinly sliced
    1 tsp. sea salt
    1 yellow onion, chopped
    1 1/2 lbs. ripe tomatoes, peeled, seeded and chopped
    2 tbsp. olive paste (available at specialty stores)
    1 tsp. black pepper

1. Bring 4 quarts of water with 1 tbsp. sea salt to boil in a large pot. Cook pasta according to directions on package. Do not over cook. It should be firm to the bite.
2. Meanwhile, heat oil in large skillet. Add onions and saute until translucent. Add garlic and tomatoes. Simmer over medium heat until liquid from tomatoes is reduced by one half. Add olive paste and basil, salt and pepper.
3. Drain pasta and toss with tomato sauce. Serve immediately.

Serves 4-6

Pasta Verde

1 lb. buckwheat noodles
6 green onions, sliced
1 bunch broccoli, cut in flowerets
1/4 cup Italian parsley, finely chopped
1 tsp. sea salt
4 oz. soft tofu
2 garlic cloves, peeled and mashed
1 lb. fresh spinach, washed and stemmed
2 tbsp. fresh basil, finely chopped
1/2 tsp. nutmeg
1 tsp. black pepper
1/2 tsp. dry mustard

1. Bring 4 quarts of water and 1 tbsp. of sea salt to boil in a large pot. Cook pasta according to directions on the package. Do not over cook. Buckwheat noodles are very fragile. Drain, reserving 1/2 cup of cooking liquid.
2. Meanwhile, place olive oil, garlic and green onions in a large sauté pan. Cook over low heat 3 to 5 minutes until onions have wilted and garlic is fragrant but not browned. Add spinach and broccoli. Toss vegetables to coat with oil. Cover and steam for 5 to 7 minutes. Uncover pan. Stir in basil, parsley, nutmeg, salt and pepper.
3. Place tofu and dry mustard in blender and blend until smooth. Add vegetables and continue to blend for 1-1/2 to 2 minutes.
4. Add hot cooking liquid to sauce in blender. Blend until smooth. Place noodles in a shallow serving bowl. Very gently toss with sauce and serve.

Serves 4-6

Artichoke Pasta

1 lb. whole wheat shells
4 medium artichokes
3 tbsp. olive oil
1 tbsp. butter
1 medium onion, thinly sliced
1 clove garlic, peeled and mashed
2 cups canned Italian plum tomatoes
1 bay leaf
1 tbsp. fresh basil, chopped
1 tsp. sea salt
1 tsp. pepper

1. Remove all tough outer leaves of artichokes. Trim and slice in half. Remove choke, then thinly slice artichoke halves lengthwise.
2. Heat oil and butter in a large skillet and add artichokes. Cook stirring constantly for 3 minutes. Add onion, garlic, tomatoes, bay leaf, basil, salt and pepper. Reduce heat to low and simmer for 25 minutes, stirring occasionally, until artichokes are tender.
3. While sauce simmers, bring 4 quarts of water and 1 tbsp. of sea salt to boil in a large pot. Add pasta and cook according to directions on package. Do not overcook. It should remain firm to the bite. Drain.
4. Place pasta in shallow serving dish. Toss with sauce and serve.

Serves 4-6

Pasta with Uncooked Tomato Sauce

1 lb. any whole grain pasta
6 medium ripe tomatoes
1 bunch basil, stemmed and chopped
4 cloves garlic, peeled and slightly crushed
3/4 cup extra virgin olive oil

1 tsp. sea salt
1 tsp. freshly ground black pepper

1. Bring a medium pan of water to a boil. Drop tomatoes into boiling water for 1-2 minutes until skins split. Core, peel and seed tomatoes. Cut into 1/4" dice. In medium bowl, mix tomatoes, basil, garlic, olive oil, salt and pepper. Cover and let sit for at least 20 minutes to blend flavors.
2. Meanwhile bring 4 quarts of water and 1 tbsp. of sea salt to boil in a large pot. Add pasta and cook according to directions on package. Do not over cook. It should remain firm to the bite. Drain.
3. Remove garlic cloves from tomato sauce. Toss with hot pasta and serve immediately.

Serves 4-6

Spinach Spaghetti with Mushrooms and Cream

1 lb. whole wheat spaghetti
6 tbsp. fresh lemon juice
1 lb. mushrooms, wiped, trimmed and sliced
4 tbsp. butter
2 cloves garlic, peeled and mashed
2 tbsp. Marsala wine (optional)
2 cups cream
2 lb. spinach, washed and stemmed
1 tsp. sea salt
1 tsp. black pepper
1/3 cup soy parmesan

1. Mix lemon juice and mushrooms together in medium bowl.
2. Melt butter in a large skillet, add garlic and Marsala. Cook for 3 minutes. Add mushrooms. Cook for 5 minutes more. Add cream and bring mixture to a boil. Stir in spinach to wilt. Add salt and pepper. Remove from heat.

3. Meanwhile, bring 4 quarts of water and 1 tbsp. sea salt to a boil in a large pot. Add pasta and cook according to directions on package. Do not over cook. It should remain firm to the bite. Drain.
4. Place pasta in shallow serving bowl. Toss gently with sauce. Serve with cheese on top.

Serves 4-6

Pasta with Garbanzos

1 lb. whole wheat penne or shells
2 15 oz. cans garbanzo beans OR 3 cups cooked garbanzos divided in half
1 tsp. fresh rosemary (2-3" sprig)
2 cloves garlic, peeled
1 tsp. sea salt
1 tsp. black pepper
2/3 cup extra virgin olive oil

1. Bring 4 quarts of water and 1 tbsp. of sea salt to boil in a large pot. Add pasta and cook according to directions on package. Do not over cook. It should remain firm to the bite. Drain, reserving cooking liquid.
2. Meanwhile, place half of garbanzo beans, rosemary, garlic, salt and pepper into food processor. Blend, adding olive oil slowly, until smooth paste is formed. Thin with cooking liquid from pasta so that sauce has the consistency of heavy cream.
3. Using a strainer, place remaining garbanzos into hot cooking liquid from pasta to warm. It need not be on the fire.
4. Place pasta in a shallow serving bowl. Toss with sauce. Gently stir remaining whole garbanzos. Serve immediately.

Serves 4-6

Fettuccine with Peas and Mint

1 lb. spinach fettuccine
1 small pinch of saffron (optional)
6 tbsp. unsalted butter
6 green onions, trimmed and sliced
1 tsp. sea salt
1 tsp. freshly ground black pepper
1 1/2 lb. fresh peas, shelled or 2 cups frozen petite peas
3 tbsp. mint leaves, finely chopped
1/4 cup soy parmesan (optional)

1. Soak saffron in a very small bowl with 2 tbsp. water
2. Combine 4 tbsp. of butter, onions, salt and pepper in a sauté pan. Cook over low heat for 15 minutes or until onions are very tender but do not allow to brown. If using fresh peas, add peas and 1/2 cup water continue to cook over low heat until peas turn bright green. If using frozen peas, add to pan and cook on low until peas are warmed enough. Stir in mint and keep warm.
3. Meanwhile, bring 4 quarts of water and 1 tbsp. of sea salt to boil in a large pot. Add fettuccine and cook according to directions on package. Do not over cook. It should be firm to the bite.
4. Combine remaining butter with saffron water in a warmed serving bowl. Remove pasta from pot leaving water dripping from strands. Toss gently with saffron butter. Gently toss with sauce. Serve with soy parmesan.

Serves 4-6

Pasta with Walnuts

1 lb. whole wheat spaghetti
3/4 cup extra virgin olive oil
2 cloves garlic, peeled and mashed
2 cups walnut halves
1 tsp. sea salt
1 tsp. freshly ground pepper
1 cup Italian parsley, roughly chopped
1 tsp. fresh orange peel (optional)

1. Place olive oil and garlic in a large sauté pan. Cook over low heat until garlic is translucent but not browned. Add walnuts, salt and pepper. Cook for 2-3 minutes to lightly brown. Keep warm.
2. Meanwhile, bring 4 quarts of water and 1 tbsp. of sea salt to a boil in large pot. Cook pasta according to directions on package. Do not over cook. Pasta should remain firm to the bite. Drain, reserving 1/2 cup of cooking liquid.
3. Place pasta in a shallow serving bowl. Toss with nut mixture, parsley, orange peel and reserved cooking liquid. Serve.

Serves 4-6

Eggplant Pasta

1 lb. whole wheat pasta shells
2 small eggplants, sliced into rounds
1/2 cup olive oil
2 cloves garlic, peeled and mashed
1 lb. fresh plum tomatoes, peeled, seeded and coarsely chopped or 1 28 oz. can Italian plum tomatoes, seeded, chopped and drained
1/2 tsp. dried red pepper flakes
1/2 tsp. black pepper
1 tbsp. fresh basil, chopped
1 tbsp. fresh parsley, chopped

1 tsp. sea salt
1/2 cup soy parmesan

1. Place sliced eggplant in colander and sprinkle with 1/2 tsp. of salt. Let drain for 30 minutes. Rinse well to remove salt and dry with a paper towel.
2. Place 1/4 cup of olive oil and garlic in a large skillet. Cook for 2-3 minutes until garlic begins to color. Add chopped tomatoes, pepper flakes, pepper, basil, parsley and remaining salt. Cook for 15 minutes until sauce thickens. Set aside and keep warm.
3. Bring 4 quarts of water and 1 tbsp. sea salt to boil in large pot. Add pasta and cook according to package directions. Do not over cook. It should be firm to bite. Drain.
4. While pasta cooks, sauté eggplant slices in remaining olive oil 3-5 minutes per side to brown evenly. Place on warm plates.
5. Gently toss cooked pasta with tomato sauce. Serve pasta over eggplant slices. Sprinkle with cheese.

Serves 4-6

VEGETABLES

It's been said a million times in a million ways and it's still true: *raw is best*. Only in it's raw state does a vegetable have every iota of nourishment nature intended. As soon as it's natural state is altered, the beloved veggie starts to loose it's nutritional power. You'll find many excellent recipes for raw vegetables in the *Salads* section of this book. But if you are going to eat *cooked* vegetables, the healthiest way will always be lightly steamed until just tender with a little lemon juice, sea salt and pepper.

Stir Fried Broccoli

>   2 bunches broccoli
>   1 tsp. sea salt
>   1 tsp. honey
>   2 tbsp. flaxseed or safflower oil
>   2 tbsp. water
>   1 tsp. cornstarch mixed with 2 tbsp. cold water

1. Separate small broccoli florets from large stems. Cut large stems thinly on the diagonal.
2. In a wok, or other large skillet, heat oil over high heat. Add broccoli and stir fry for 2 minutes. Add salt, water and honey. Toss well. Cover and continue cooking for 2 minutes longer, stirring once. Add cornstarch mixture. Toss well. Cook 1 minute more and serve immediately.

Serves 4-6

Spring Greens

8 cups greens, such as turnips, beets, chard, spinach or a mixture which could include watercress and dandelions as well
2 tbsp. flaxseed or safflower oil
1 large onion, sliced thinly
1 1/2 tbsp. molasses
3 tbsp. apple cider vinegar

1. Place washed greens in a steamer. Steam until just wilted. Chop greens coarsely with a knife.
2. Heat oil in skillet over medium heat. Add onions, cooking until translucent but not brown. Meanwhile, mix molasses and vinegar together in a small bowl. Add to onion mixture, stirring well. Add greens. Toss to mix well and serve.

Serves 4

Spinach with Currants and Nuts

6 bunches spinach, washed and stems removed
2/3 cup currants, soaked in warm water for 30 minutes and well drained
1/4 cup olive oil
1/2 cup pine nuts
1/2 tsp. sea salt
1/2 tsp. black pepper

1. Place spinach in a steamer and steam until just wilted. Squeeze out extra moisture.
2. Heat oil over medium heat in a fireproof casserole or heavy skillet. Add pine nuts and cook over medium heat until they begin to color. Add currants and stir well. Add

spinach, salt and pepper and heat through. Serve immediately.

Serves 4-6

Green Beans with Garlic

4 tbsp. olive oil
3 cloves garlic, peeled and sliced
1 lb. green beans, strings removed
1 tsp. sea salt
1/2 tsp. black pepper
3 cups whole grain bread crumbs

1. Heat oil in a large skillet over medium heat. Add garlic cloves, cooking until translucent, then add beans, salt and pepper and stir to coat with oil.
2. Increase heat when beans begin to turn color. Toss in bread crumbs, stirring briskly so that they do not stick and burn on bottom of pan. Transfer to warmed serving dish and serve.

Serves 4

Crusty herbed Cauliflower

1 large cauliflower
1 tbsp. egg replacer mixed with 4 tbsp. water
1/2 tsp. sea salt
1 cup whole grain bread crumbs
1/4 cup fresh basil, chopped
1/4 cup fresh parsley, chopped
3 tbsp. whole wheat flour
1 tsp. spike
2 tbsp. melted butter

1. Cut cauliflower into florets. Place in steamer and steam 10-12 minutes until just tender.
2. Meanwhile, mix together egg replacer and salt in a small bowl. In a separate bowl, mix together bread crumbs, basil and parsley.
3. Toss florets with flour and spike to dust lightly. Dip each into egg replacer mixture, then bread crumb mixture. Place on non-stick or oiled baking sheet. Drizzle with melted butter. Bake in preheated 350° oven for 20-25 minutes until golden and crispy.

Serves 6

Japanese Snow Peas

2 tbsp. sesame oil
1 lb. mushrooms, brushed clean with a vegetable brush then thinly sliced
1 lb. snow peas, trimmed
1 tbsp. tamari soy sauce

1. Heat oil in wok or large skillet over high heat. Add mushrooms and stir fry for 2 minutes. Add peas and cook 1 minute more, just to turn the color of the peas. They should be just barely heated through and very crispy. Add tamari soy sauce, mix well and serve.

Serves 4

Baked Potatoes with Leeks

4 large baking potatoes
4 tbsp. butter
2 leeks, split, washed and finely sliced
1 tsp. sea salt
1 tsp. black pepper
1/3 cup cream
1 tbsp. any fresh herb, finely chopped

2 tbsp. soy parmesan cheese

1. Bake potatoes in a 400° oven for 50 minutes or until soft when pierced with a fork. Allow to cool enough to handle. Split potatoes in half lengthwise.
2. Meanwhile, heat butter in a medium skillet. Add leeks and cook over low heat until leeks are very soft and translucent. Season with salt and pepper.
3. Scoop out the pulp of the potatoes, careful not to break the shells. Place pulp in mixing bowl, breaking it up with a fork or whisk. Add cream and beat until smooth. Fold in leek mixture and fresh herbs. Refill potato skins, sprinkle tops with cheese and put under broiler for 5 minutes or until browned.

Serves 4

Baked Tomatoes

8 medium tomatoes
4 cloves garlic, peeled and slivered
1 1/2 cups whole wheat sourdough bread crumbs
2 tbsp. fresh parsley, chopped
1/2 cup olive oil

1. Remove hard core from tomatoes with tip of knife. Slice off tops. Push garlic slivers down into sections of each tomato and place in shallow baking dish.
2. Mix crumbs with parsley, salt and pepper. Lightly stuff centers of tomatoes, piling bread crumbs on top of each. Drizzle with oil. Bake in preheated 400° oven for 20-25 minutes until tops are golden and tomatoes are soft. Serve warm or break on top of nest of freshly cooked pasta.

Serves 4

Stir Fry Asparagus

2 lb. asparagus, tough end trimmed off
2 tbsp. safflower oil
3 tbsp. soy sauce
1 tbsp. lemon juice
1/2 tsp. sea salt
1/2 tsp. black pepper

1. Cut asparagus into thin diagonal slices. Place in steamer and steam just until asparagus turns bright green. Remove from steamer basket at once.
2. Heat oil in wok or large skillet. Add asparagus, soy sauce, lemon juice, salt and pepper. Toss well to coat. Cook for 1 minute. Do not over cook. Serve.

Serves 4

GRAINS AND LEGUMES

The primary source of protein of the Livingston Foundation Program is grains and legumes, since dairy products, with the exception of cream and butter, are disallowed. For complicated chemical reasons, any legume by itself is incomplete as a protein source, hence must be complemented with a grain.

Bean Polenta

> 2 cups dried red or navy beans, soaked overnight and drained
> 1 tbsp. red wine vinegar
> 1 1/2 tsp. prepared mustard
> 1 tsp. black pepper
> 3 tbsp. fresh lemon juice
> 1 tbsp. molasses
> 1 tbsp. butter
> 2 tsp. sea salt
> drinking water for soaking beans

1. Place beans in a pot and cover with cold drinking water. Bring water to a boil, then simmer, adding just enough water to keep beans covered for two hours.
2. Pour beans into a sieve and press them through. Place resulting pulp in a large skillet with lemon juice, molasses, vinegar, butter, mustard, salt and pepper. Gently heat for 5 to 7 minutes. Serve.

Serves 4-6

Kidney Beans with Walnut Sauce

1 cup dried kidney beans, soaked overnight and drained, <u>OR</u> 2 cups canned kidney beans heated (begin recipe at step 2)
1 tbsp. red wine vinegar, mixed with 3 tbsp. water
2 tbsp. fresh parsley
2 tsp. sea salt
1/3 cup walnut pieces
1 garlic clove, peeled and mashed
1/4 tsp. cayenne pepper
2 tbsp. onion, finely chopped
2 tbsp. Cilanto, or 1/2 tsp. Ground coriander, finely chopped
drinking water for beans

1. Place beans in a pot, cover them with drinking water and cook uncovered for 2 hours until beans are tender but still intact. Drain and toss with salt.
2. In a mortar, or food processor, pound or process walnuts with garlic and cayenne. Place in a small glass mixing bowl. Stir in vinegar/water mixture until well blended. Add walnut paste, onions, coriander and parsley to beans. Mix well being careful not to bruise beans. May be chilled before serving.

Serves 4

Lima Bean Casserole

2/3 cup dried lima beans, soaked overnight and drained
2 tbsp. olive oil
1 large green bell pepper, seeded and diced
2 ribs celery, diced
1 large onion, chopped
1 clove garlic, peeled and mashed
1/2 cup raisins
1 1/2 tbsp. sesame seeds
3/4 cup soy "jack" cheese, grated
drinking water for beans

1. Place beans in a pot, cover them with cold water. Bring water to boil, then simmer, adding just enough water to keep beans covered for two hours or until tender. Drain, reserve cooking liquid.
2. In a large skillet heat oil. Add green pepper, celery, onion and garlic. Cook over medium heat 10 minutes or until tender. Stir pepper/onion mixture into beans, 1 1/2 cup cooking liquid (add water if necessary), raisins and sesame seeds and half of the cheese.
3. Turn mixture into a large oiled casserole. Bake in a preheated 375° oven for 25 minutes. Sprinkle on remaining cheese, return to oven for 10 minutes to allow cheese to melt and form a bubbly crust.

Serves 4-6

Bohemian Yellow Peas

2 cups dried yellow peas, soaked overnight and drained
1 sprig fresh thyme or 1/2 tsp. dried thyme
1 bay leaf
3 whole cloves
4 peppercorns
2 small onions, thinly sliced
1 carrot, scrubbed and chopped finely
6 cups drinking water
6 tbsp. butter
3 tbsp. dry whole bread crumbs sautéed in 2 tsp. butter
1 tsp. sea salt
1/2 tsp. black pepper

1. Wrap the thyme, bay leaf, cloves, peppercorns and a few slices of the onion in a double layer of cheesecloth. Tie securely. Place the seasoning bag, the carrot and peas in a large pot with the 6 cups of water. Bring to boil. Cook for 1 1/2 hours until peas are soft. Discard the seasoning bag. Drain peas.

2. Melt butter in a large skillet. Add remaining onions and cook over medium heat until they are translucent but not brown. Set aside.
3. Coat a 6-cup baking dish with remaining butter. Coat with 2 tbsp. dry bread crumbs. Season the peas with salt and pepper. Place in baking dish. Top with sautéed onions, then cover with remaining 1 tbsp. bread crumbs. Bake in a preheated 375° oven for 15 minutes to warm through and crisp top. Serve immediately.

Serves 6

Tofu Stew

1/2 cup safflower oil
2 onions, sliced
2 cloves garlic
2 carrots, scrubbed and coarsely chopped
1/2 lb. green cabbage, coarsely chopped
2 tofu cakes, sliced into 16 equal pieces
1/2 lb. green beans, trimmed
1 cup drinking water
1/2 cup soy sauce

1. Heat oil in large casserole. Add onions and garlic. Cook until soft but not browned. Add carrots and cabbage. Sauté for 1 minute more.
2. Add tofu, green beans, water and soy sauce. Gently bring mixture to boil for 15-20 minutes, until the juices thicken slightly.

Serves 6

Lentils with Lemon & Chard

1 1/2 cups dried lentils
drinking water for cooking lentils
2 1/2 lb. chard, stems removed but a few reserved and chopped with the leaves
3/4 cup olive oil
1 medium onion, chopped
1/3 cup celery, chopped
2 cloves garlic, peeled and mashed
1 tsp. whole wheat pastry flour
3/4 cup fresh lemon juice
1 1/2 tsp. sea salt
1 tsp. black pepper

1. In a large pot, cook lentils in enough water to cover for 15-20 minutes until tender. Add chard and cook another 10 minutes.
2. Meanwhile, heat oil in a skillet. Add onions, celery and garlic. Sauté until translucent. Stir in flour and lemon juice. Add this mixture to the lentils. Season with salt and pepper. Simmer 10-15 minutes until sauce has thickened.

Serves 6

Brown Rice with Almonds & Mushrooms

1 cup long grained brown rice
2 1/2 cups vegetable broth
3 stalks celery, chopped
1/2 cup almonds, slivered
1/2 tsp. dried marjoram or rosemary
2 tsp. sea salt
1 large onion, diced
1/4 cup cold pressed vegetable oil
1 tbsp. fresh sage, or 1 tsp. rubbed dry
1/2 lb. mushrooms, brushed clean with a vegetable brush and sliced

1. Combine rice, sea salt and broth in a heavy duty pan. Bring to a boil and stir. Cover and reduce heat to a low simmer for 50 minutes or until rice is tender and liquid is absorbed.
2. Meanwhile, sauté onion and celery in oil until translucent but not browned. Add almonds and continue to cook for 3 minutes stirring frequently so the nuts do not burn. Add herbs and mushrooms. Continue to sauté until mushrooms are wilted. Combine with rice and mix well.
3. This dish may be kept warm in a 350 F. oven.

Serves 4

Carrot and Wild Rice Casserole

1 tbsp. flaxseed or safflower oil
1 large onion, chopped
4 cups cooked wild rice
2 cups carrot, finely chopped
1/4 cup pecans
1 tsp. sea salt
1 cup cream
1 1/2 tsp. egg replacer mixed in 2 tbsp. water

1. Heat oil in skillet. Add onions, cooking over medium heat until onions are translucent but not browned.
2. Add wild rice, carrots, pecans and salt to onions. Mix well.
3. Combine cream and egg replacer in a small bowl. Fold into rice mixture.
4. Turn mixture into a buttered 2 quart casserole. Bake, covered, in preheated 350° oven for 30 minutes. Remove cover and stir well. Continue baking for 10 minutes more until rice is firm.

Serves 4-6

Syrian Cracked Wheat Banadoora

1/4 cup extra virgin olive oil
1/2 cup onion, chopped
1 cup mushrooms, brushed clean with a vegetable brush and sliced
1 1/2 cups cracked wheat
2 1/2 cups vegetable broth
1/2 cup tomato sauce
1 tsp. sea salt
1/2 tsp. black pepper
1 tbsp. lemon juice
1 tsp. fresh dill or 1/2 tsp. dried
1/2 tsp. fresh mint, chopped
1/2 tsp. cumin (optional)

1. Heat oil in large skillet. Add onions. Cook until translucent but not browned. Add mushrooms, continue cooking over medium heat until all liquid has been absorbed.
2. Add cracked wheat, broth, tomato sauce, salt and pepper. Cook, covered, over very low heat for 15-20 minutes until liquid is absorbed. Stir in lemon juice, dill, mint and cumin. Serve warm or at room temperature.

Serves 4-6

DESSERTS

Let's face it—a lot of diets can bore you to tears and take all of the joy out of dining. We have taken great pains to develop a variety of healthful yet tasty for the end of your meal. The best and easiest dessert will always be fresh fruit in season and served attractively.

Dried Fruit Compote

    1 cup dried apples, unsulphured
    1 cup prunes, unsulphured
    8 cups drinking water
    1/2 cup sunflower seeds
    1 cup whipped cream sweetened with 1 tbsp. apple juice
    1 cup dried apricots, unsulphured
    1/2 cup golden raisins
    2 cinnamon sticks
    1/4 cup almonds, slivered and toasted

1. In a large sauce pan, combine all fruits, sunflower seeds and cinnamon sticks with water. Bring to a boil. Lower heat, cover the pan with a lid and simmer slowly for 45 minutes. Compote may be served hot, room temperature or chilled.
2. Top with almonds and whipped cream.

Serves 4-6

Fruit Sorbet

2 cups frozen fruit or berries
tbsp. fresh lime juice

1. Place fruit in juicer with blank blade instead of screen. Blend in lime juice. Press puree through sieve placed over fruit cups and serve.
Serves 4-6

Frozen Peach Delight

1 cup apple juice
1/2 cup almond butter
1 tsp. vanilla
2 cups fresh peaches, frozen
3 bananas, cut into pieces and frozen

1. Place juice, almond butter and vanilla in blender. Blend until smooth. Add frozen fruit 1/2 cup at a time ending with the frozen bananas. This will thicken the mixture. Pour into chilled parfait glasses or custard cups. Serve at once.
Makes 4-6 servings

Strawberry Banana Custard

4 ripe bananas, cut into pieces
1 tbsp. lime juice
2 cups strawberries, sliced or 1-16 oz. package frozen strawberries, thawed
2 cups drinking water
1/2 cup quick cooking tapioca

1. Place bananas and lime juice in blender. Blend until smooth. Place in medium sauce pan. Add berries and their

juice, tapioca and water. Mix well. Let stand for 5 minutes. Heat fruit mixture to boiling, stirring constantly. Remove from heat. Let stand for 20-25 minutes to thicken. Serve in custard cups. May be topped with tofu cream and nuts if desired.

Serves 6

Cherry Pudding

5 tbsp. arrowroot
2 cups drinking water
1/2 tsp. raw honey
1 tbsp. cherry juice concentrate
1 tsp. lemon peel, finely grated

1. Stir arrowroot into 1/2 cup cold water.
2. Bring remaining water to boil in medium sauce pan. Add arrowroot mixture, stirring over medium-high heat for 5 minutes until mixture clears and thickens.
3. Remove from heat and add honey, cherry juice and lemon peel. Cool in refrigerator at least 1/2 hour until set.

Serves 4

Carob Oatmeal Cookies

1/2 cup pitted dates
1/2 cup rolled oats
1/2 tsp. sea salt
1 tsp. vanilla
2 tbsp. butter
1 cup buckwheat
3 ripe bananas
1/2 cup carob chips

1. Process dates and butter together in a food processor. Place in a small sauce pan and cook over a low heat for 3 to 5 minutes until mixture is well blended. Cool.
2. Preheat oven to 375°. Place oats in food processor. Process to form oat flour. Combine in medium bowl with buckwheat flour and salt. Set aside.
3. In a large mixing bowl, mash bananas until smooth. Blend in date butter and vanilla until smooth. Stir in flour mixture. Fold in carob chips.
4. Using a mixing spoon, make 1" mounds on non-stick baking sheet. Bake 12 to 15 minutes until lightly browned.

Makes 2 dozen cookies

Bee-Licious Bars

1 cup cashew butter
1 cup raw honey
1 cup carob powder
1 cup sunflower seeds
2/3 cup granola
1/2 cup almonds, chopped
1/2 cup raisins, preferably golden
1/2 cup unsweetened coconut, shredded
4 tbsp. bee pollen granules
1 tsp. sesame seeds

1. In a medium sauce pan, heat cashew butter and honey over low heat, stirring until smooth. Remove from heat.
2. Stir in remaining ingredients. Press into an 8" square baking pan. Chill and cut into squares.

Makes 16 squares

Tofu Cheesecake

2 cups granola
1/4 cup apple juice
48 oz. tofu
4 tbsp. raw honey
1 cup soy milk
1/2 cup tahini
2 tsp. fresh lemon juice
1 tsp. vanilla
1/2 tsp. sea salt

1. Mix granola with apple juice. Press into the bottom of an 8" or 9" springform pan. Bake at 400° for 8-10 minutes. Cool
2. Meanwhile, drain tofu and press to remove excess liquid. Place in blender with honey, soy milk, tahini, lemon juice, vanilla and sea salt. Blend until smooth. Pour filling into springform pan. Bake at 325° for 30 minutes. When center of cake is firm, turn off heat and let cake remain in oven for another 30 minutes. Allow to cool then refrigerate overnight. Flavor is best when allowed to rest for 2 days.

Serves 12

Tofu Cream

8 oz. soft tofu
1/2 cup rice malt syrup
1 tbsp. cold pressed safflower oil
1 tsp. vanilla
1/8 tsp. sea salt

1. Drain tofu in strainer for 15 minutes. Combine all ingredients in blender and process until smooth. Options include substituting citrus rind or other extract for vanilla.

Makes 1 1/2 cups

Whipped Cream

1 cup heavy cream
1 tbsp. honey
1 tsp. vanilla

1. In a chilled mixing bowl, beat cream until thickened to form soft peaks. Add honey and vanilla. Continue beating until stiff peaks form. Do not over beat, as cream quickly turns to butter.

Makes 1 cup

BIBLIOGRAPHY

Acevedo, H., Slifkin, M., Poucher, G.R. and Pardo, M., *Immunohistochemical localization of a chorio-gonadotropin-like protein in bacteria isolated from cancer patients*, Cancer, 41: 1217-29, 1978.

Albeaux-Fernet, M., *Syndromes hormonaux ectopicques*, Sem. Hop., Paris, 49:4, 245-56, 1973.

Alexander-Jackson, E., *A specific type of microorganism isolated from animal and human cancer: Bacteriology of the orgnism*, Proc. VIth Cong. Microbiol., (Sect. VIIA), Growth, 19: 37-51, 1954.

Alexander-Jackson, E., *Mycoplasma (PPLO) isolated from Rous sarcoma virus*, Growth, 9: 219-228, 1966.

Alexander-Jackson, E., *Ultraviolet spectrogramic microscope studies of Rous sarcoma virus cultured in cell free medium*, Ann. N.Y. Acad. Sci., (Art. 2), 174: 765-81, 1970.

Acevedo, H.F., Campbell-Acevedo, E. and Kloos, W.E., *Expression of human choriogonadotropin-like material in coagulase negative Staphylococci species*, Inf. & Imm., 50: 860-68, 1986.

Affronti, L.F., Grow, F. and Begell, F., *Characterization of bacterial tumor isolates*, Fed. Proc., 1043, 1975.

Beard, J., The Enzyme Treatment of Cancer. London: Chatto and Windus, 1911.

Backus, B.T. and Affronti, L.F., *Tumor-associated bacteria capable of producing a human choriogonadotropin-like substance*. Inf. & Imm., 32: 1211-15, 1981.

Braunstein, G.D., Vaitukaitus, J.L., Carbone, P.P. and Ross, G.T., *Ectopic production of human chorionic gonadotropin by neoplasms.* Ann. Intern. Med., 78: 39-45, 1973.

Busch, W., *Niederngeinischen Gesellschaft fur Nature-end Reilkunde in Bonn. Aus der Sitzung der Medizenischen Sektion* Vol 13. Nov. 1987. Ber. Klin. Wschr. 5: 137-9, 1868.

Cantwell, A.R., Kelso, D.W. and Rowe, L., *Hypodermitis sclerodermiformis and unusual acid fast bacteria.* Arch. Dermatol., 115: 449-452, 1979.

Cantow, M.J.R., and Johnson, J.E., J. App. Pol. Sci., II: 1851, 1967

Clark, G.A., *Successful culturing of Glover's cancer organism and development of metastasizing tumors in animals produced by cultures from human malignancy.* Proc. Cong. of Microb., Rome, Italy, 1953.

Cohen, H. and Stampp, A., *Bacterial synthesis of a substance similar to human chorionic gonadotropin.* Proc. Soc. Exper. Biol. Med., 152: 408-10, 1976.

Cianciolo, G.J., *Antiinflamatory proteins associated with human murine neoplasms*, Biochem. Biophys. Acta, 865: 69-82, 1986.

Cassileth, B.R., Luck, E.J., Guerry, D., Blake, A.D., Walsh, W.P., Kascius, L. and Schultz, D.J., *Survival and quality of life among patients receiving unproven as compared with conventional cancer therapy.* New Eng. J. Med., 324: 1180-85.

Coley, W.R., *Contributions to the knowledge of sarcoma.* Ann. Surg., 14: 199-220, 1891.

Diller, I.C., *Tumor incidence in ICR/albino and C57/B 16JN/cr male mice injected organisms cultured from mouse malignant tissues.* Growth, 38: 507-17, 1974.

Diller, I.C., *Growth and morphological variability of three similar strains of intermittently acid-fast organism isolated from mouse and human malignant tissues.* Growth, 26: 181-208, 1965.

Domingue, G.J., Schlegel, J.U. and Woody, H.E., *Naked bacteria in human blood. A novel concept for etiology of certain kidney diseases.* Ann. Meeting of Amer. Soc. for Microb., 2: 2, 1976.

Domingue, G.J., Acevedo, H.N., Powell, J.E. and Stevens, V.C., *Antibodies to bacterial vaccines demonstrating specificity for human choriogonadotropin (HCG) and immunochemical detection of HCG-like factor in subcellular bacterial fractions.* Inf. & Immunology., 53: 95-98, 1986.

DeVita, V.T., *Progress in Cancer Research.* Cancer, 51: 2401-09, 1983.

Davis, M.J., Purcell, A.H. and Thompson, S.V., *Pierce's disease of grapevines, isolation of the causal bacterium.* Science, 199: 75-8, 1978.

Dilman, V.M., Golubev, V.N. and Krylova, N.V., *Dissociation of hormonal and antigenic activity of luteinizing hormone excreted in endometrial carcinoma patients (endogenous anahormones).* Amer. J. of Obstetrics Gynecol., 7:115, 966-71, 1973.

Ellouz, F., Adam, A., Ciorbaru, R. and Lederer, E., *Minimal structural requirements for adjuvant activity of bacterial peptidoglycan derivatives.* Biochem.-Biophys. Res. Communication. 66: 1316, 1975.

Fidler, I.J. and Poste, G., *The cellular Heterogenicity of malignant neoplasms. Implications for adjuvant chemotherapy.* Semin. Oncology. 12: 207-22, 1985.

Fonti, C.J., Eziopatogenese del cancro, Amadeo Nicola, Milan, Italy, 1958.

Gerlach, F., <u>Krebs and obligator pilzparasitismus</u>, Urban and Schwartzenberg, Vienna, Austria, 1948.

Glover, T.J., *The bacteriology of cancer*, <u>Canada Lancet Pract.</u>, 74: 92-111, 1930.

Glover, T.J., Scott, M.J., Loudon, J. and McCormack, M., *Study of Rous chicken sarcoma No 1*, <u>Canada Lancet Pract.</u>, 66-49, 1926.

Gurdon, J.B., *Transplanted nuclei and cell differentiation.* <u>Science America</u>, 219: 24-35, 1968.

Inoue, S., Singer, M. and Huntchinson, J., *Causative agent of a spontaneously originatin visceral tumor of the Newt Trinitus.* <u>Nature</u>, 205: 408-9, 1965.

Kellen, J.A., Kolin, A. and Acevedo, H.F., Acevedo effect of antibodies to choriogonadotropin in malignant growth. I. Rat 3230 AC Mammary Adenocarcinoma cancer, 49: 2300.

Kellen, J.A., Kolin, A. and Mirakian, H.F., *Effects of antibodies to choriogonadotropin in malignant growth.* II. Solid transplantable rat tumors. <u>Cancer Immunotherapy</u> 13: 2-4, 1982.

Koide, S.S., Cohen, H. and Maruo, T., *Studies of choriogonadotropin from a microorganism.* <u>Endo. Soc.</u>, 1979.

Lange, P.H., Hakala, T.R. and Fraley, E.E., *Supression of an antitumor lymphocyte mediated cytotoxicity by human gonadotropins.* <u>J. Urology</u>, 115: 95-8, 1976.

Leyton, A.S. and Leyton, H., *Observations on the aetilogy of sarcoma in the rat.* <u>Lancet</u>, i: 513, 1916.

Livingston, V., Wheeler, W.C. and Alexander-Jackson, E., *A specific type of organism cultivated from malignancy; Bacteriology and proposed classifications.* <u>Ann. N.Y. Acad. Sci</u>, (Art. 2), 174: 636-54, 1970.

Livingston, V., W-C. Livingston, A.M., Alexander-Jackson, E. and Wolter, G.H., *Toxic fractions obtained from tumor isolates and related clinical implications*. Ann. N.Y. Acad. Sci. (Art. 2), 174: 675-89, 1970.

Livingston, V., W-C. and Livingston, A.M., *Demonstration of Progenitor Cryptocides in the blood of patients with collagen and neoplastic diseases*. Trans. N.Y. Acad. Sci., (Series II, No. 5), 34: 433-53, 1972.

Livingston-Wheeler, V. and Majnarich, J.J., (Oct. 18, 1983), *Method of preparing a purified extraction residue fraction and its use in stimulating the immune response*. U.S. Patent 4,410,510.

MacPherson, I., *Reversion of hamster cells transformed by Rous sarcoma virus*, Science, 148: 1731, 1965.

Mankiewicz, E., *Antigenic components shared by bacteriophages and phase hosts: Mycobacteria, corynebacteria and hela cells*. Growth, 29: 125-39, 1965.

Marua, G., Cohen, H., Segal, S.J. and Koide, S.S., *Production of choriogonadotropin-like factors by a microorganism*. Proc. Natl. Acad. Sci. USA, 76: 662-6, 1979.

Mazet, G., Presence *d'elements alcooloacido resistants dans les moelles leucemiquies et les moelles non-lecemiques*, La Semaine des Hopitaus (Medicine dans le Monde), 38 e Anee, 1-2:35, 1962.

Merser, C., Sinay, P. and Adam, A., *Total synthesis and Adjuvant Activity of Bacterial Peptidoglycan derivatives*. Biochem. Biophys. Res. Commun., 66: 1316, 1975.

Meyers, A.R., Sanchez, D., Elwell, L.P. and Falkow, S., A simple agarose gel electrophoretic method for the identification and characterization of plasmid desoxyribonucleic acid. J. Bacteriol. 127: 1529-37, 1976.

Midgley, A.R., Endocrinology, 79: 10, 1966.

Mousselon-Canet, M., *Analogs of abscisic acid and or dormancy hormone structure activity.* C.R. Acad. Sci., Paris, 270: 1936-9. 1970.

Nakamura, S., Sakurada, S., Salahuddin, S.J., Osada, Y., Tanaka, N.G., Sakamoto, N., Sekiguchi, M. and Gallo, R.C., *Inhibition of development of Kaposiís sarcoma-related lesions by a bacterial cell wall complex.* Science, 255: 1437-40, 1992.

Nazum, J.W., *Experimental production of metastasizing carcinoma inbreast of dog and primary epithelioma in man by repeated inoculation of micrococcus isolated from human breast cancer.* Surg. Gyn. Obstet., 11: 343-52, 1925.

Oldham, R.K., *Biotherapy: general principles.* Principles of Cancer Biotherapy, pp 1-20, 1987.

Pease, P.E., *Tolerated infection with the sub-bacterial phase of listeria,* Nature, 215: 936-8, 1967.

Rosen, S.W., Weintraub, B.D., Vaitukaitis, J.L., Sussman, H.H., Herschman, J.M. and Muggia, F.M., *Placental proteins and their subunits as tumor markers.* Ann. Intern. Med. 82: 71-83, 1975.

Rosenthal, S.R., *The present status of the role of the immune system in cancer and leukemia and proposal for prophylactic vaccination with BCG against neoplasia,* Cancer Cytology, 8-17, 1976.

Scott, M.J., *Clinical experiences with carcinoma anti-toxin,* J. Cancer, 3: 1-6, 1926.

Siebert, F.B., Farrelly, F.K. and Shepard, C.C., *DMSO and other combatants against bacteria isolated from leukemia,* Ann. N.Y. Acad. Sci., 141: 175-201, 1967.

Seibert, F.B., Farrelly, F.K., Davis, R.L. and Richmond, I.S., *Morphological, biological and immunological studies on isolates from tumors and leukemic bloods*. Ann. N.Y. Acad. Sci., ((Art. 2), 174: 690-728, 1970.

Seibert, F.B., Baker, A., Dierking, J., Abadal, R. and Davis, R., *Decrease in spontaneous tumors by vaccinating C3H mice with an homologous bacterial vaccine*. Int. Res. Comm. System 1:53, 1973.

Seibert, F.B. and Davis, R.L., *Delay in tumor development induced with a bacterial vaccine*. Reticulo-endothelial Soc. J., 21: 279-82, 1977.

Seibert, F.B., Yeomans, F., Baker, J., Davis, R. and Diller, I.C., *Bacteria in Tumors*. Trans. N.Y. Acad. Sci., 34: 504-33, 1972.

Stewart-Tull, D.E.S., *Immunologically important constituents of mycobacteria: adjuvants in the Biology of the mycobacteria*, Vol. 2, (Eds. Ratledge, C. & Stanford, J.) Academic Press, pp 3-84, 1983.

Stewart-Tull, D.E.S., Immunopotentiating Conjugates Vaccine, 3: 40-5, 1985.

Studer, H., Staub, J.J. and Wyss, F., Schweiz Med. Wschr., Nr. 13, 101: 446-7, 1971.

Vaitukaitis, J.L., *Immunological and physical characterization of human Chorionic Gonadotropin (HCG) secreted by tumors*. J. Clin. Endocrinol. Metab. 37: 505-14, 1973.

Vaitukaitis, J.L. and Ebersole, E.R., *Evidence for altered synthesis of Chorionic Gonadotrpin in gestational trophoblastic tumors*. J. Clin. Endocrinol. Metab., 42: 1048-55, 1976.

Villequez, E.J., Le parasitisme latent des cellules du sang chez l'homme, en particulier dans le sang le cancereux, Maloine, Paris, France, 1955.

Waldenstrom, J.G., *Maladies of derepression, monoclonal derepression of protein froming templates*, Schweiz, Med. Wschr., 100: 2197-2206. 1970.

Wilson, T.S., McDowell, E.M., McIntyre, K.R. and Trump, B.F., *Elaboration of human chorionic gonadotropin by lung tumors*, Arch. Pathol. Lab. Med., 105: 169, 1981.

Wuerthele-Caspe, V. (Livingston-Wheeler) and Alexander-Jackson, E., *An experimental biologic approach to the treatment of neoplastic disease.* J. Amer. Med. Wom. Assn., 20: 858-66, 1965.

Wuerthele-Caspe, V. (Livingston-Wheeler), Alexander-Jackson, E., Anderson, J.A., Hillier, J., Allen, R.M. and Smith, L.W., *Cultural properties and pathogenicity of certain microorganisms obtained from various proliferative and neoplastic diseases.* Amer. J. Med. Sci., 220: 628-46, 1959.

Wuerthele-Caspe, V. (Livingston-Wheeler), Alexander-Jackson, E. and Smith, L.W., *Some aspects of the microbiology of cancer.* J. Amer. Med. Wom. Assn., 8: 7-12, 1953

Wuerthele-Caspe, V. (Livingston-Wheeler) and Allen, R.M., *Microorganisms associated with neoplasms.* N.Y. Microscopical Soc. (Bull.2), 2-31, 1948.

SUGGESTED READINGS

Canales, Ana Maria, *The Cookbook*, San Diego, California: The Livingston Foundation, 1996.

de Kruif, Paul, *Microbe Hunters*, San Diego, New York, & London: Harcourt Brace & Company, 1926.

Diamond, W. John, MD and Cowden, W. Lee MD with Goldberg, Burton, *An Alternative Medicine Definitive Guide to Cancer*, Tiburon, California: Future Medicine Publishing, Inc. 1997.

Fink, John M., *Third Opinion*, Garden City Park, New York: Avery Publishing Group (now Penguin Putnam Publishing), 1997.

Hess, David J., PhD, *Can Bacteria Cause Cancer?*, New York University Press, New York & London, 1997

Netterberg, Robert E., DDS and Taylor, Robert T., *The Cancer Conspiracy*: New York, New York: Pinnacle Books (now Penguin Books), 1981.

Thomas, Lewis, MD, *The Lives of a Cell: Notes of a Biology Watcher*, New York, New York: The Viking Press, 1974.

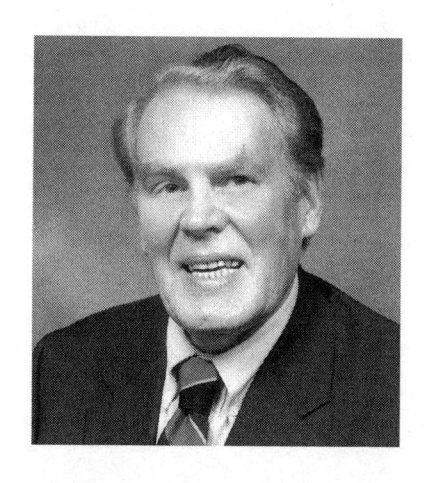

ABOUT THE AUTHOR

Arthur Douglass Alexander graduated from Case Institute of Technology where he majored in Chemical Engineering and Engineering Management. He later completed graduate studies in Biochemistry at Cornell Medical College (Sloan-Kettering Biosciences Division). Alexander has over 35 years experience in chemical and biological research and management activities. He served as assistant to Dr. C. Chester Stock, Scientific Director of Sloan-Kettering Institute for Cancer Research in New York where he managed the Experimental Chemotherapy program before being appointed Associate Director of the Children's Cancer Research Foundation in Boston. He next worked with Dr. Edwin Land at

Polaroid Corporation on the development of Polaroid color film. This was followed by a position as Senior Scientist with NASA. During this time Alexander met and became scientific advisor to Dr. Virginia Livingston. Currently on the Board of Directors at the Livingston Foundation for Cancer Research and Related Diseases, he has been appointed Vice President, Assistant to the President, Chief Operating Officer, and Scientific Director of the Foundation and the Livingston Foundation Medical Center in San Diego. Alexander is a member of many professional associations, including the New York Academy of Sciences, the American Chemical Society, Royal Society of Chemists and is a Fellow of the American Institute of Chemists. He has written many scientific papers and in 1998 authored <u>The Curious Man, The Life and Works of Dr. Hans A. Nieper, MD</u> of Hannover, Germany, a leading clinical researcher and proponent of complementary medicine in the treatment of chronic diseases.